Clinical Skills
for Medical Students
A Hands-on Guide
2nd Edition

Ian Bickle MB BCh BAO (Hons)
Senior House Officer
Royal Victoria Hospital
Belfast

Paul Hamilton BSc (Hons) MB BCh BAO (Hons)
Senior House Officer
Belfast City Hospital
Belfast

Barry Kelly MD, FRCS, FRCR, FFRRCSI
Consultant Radiologist
Royal Victoria Hospital
Belfast

David McCluskey MD, FRCP, FRCPI
Head of Department of Medicine
Queen's University Belfast
Belfast

D0474122

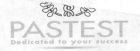

PASTEST
Dedicated to your success

First published 2001
Second Edition 2005

ISBN: 1 904627 43 9

A catalogue record for this book is available from the British Library.

The information contained within this book was obtained by the authors from reliable sources. However, while every effort has been made to ensure its accuracy, no responsibility for loss, damage or injury occasioned to any person acting or refraining from action as a result of information contained herein can be accepted by the publishers or authors.

PasTest Revision Books and Intensive Courses

PasTest has been established in the field of postgraduate medical education since 1972, providing revision books and intensive study courses for doctors preparing for their professional examinations.

Books and courses are available for the following specialties:
MRCP Part 1 and 2, MRCPCH Part 1 and 2, MRCGP, MRCPsych, MRCS, MRCOG, DRCOG, DCH, FRCA, PLAB.

For further details contact:
PasTest, Haig Road, Knutsford, Cheshire WA16 8DX
Tel: 01565 752000   Fax: 01565 650264
www.pastest.co.uk   enquiries@pastest.co.uk

Text and illustrations prepared by Cox Design Partnership, Oxon
Printed and bound in Europe by The Alden Group

CONTENTS — v —

This book on practical clinical skills has been carefully produced with the medical student in mind. It is for this reason that we hope you find it applicable and focused to your needs. Our intentions were to produce something that students would turn to on a regular basis because it is easy to follow, concise and useful for everyday practice.

It is doubtful whether anyone could develop their own clinical skills without instruction and demonstration from more experienced colleagues. This is why we would encourage you to ask someone if you don't understand a particular test or aspect of an examination. We have sought, and will continue to seek, the advice and skills of more senior medics. For this reason it is only proper that we acknowledge all those who have instructed and taught us across Northern Ireland's hospitals. A special thanks goes to all the staff at the Clinical Skills Centre at Belfast City Hospital, a comforting and ideal learning environment from the earliest days of our medical education.

The clarity and readability of this text owes much to Mary McCaffery and Glen Clarke, who constructively criticised all aspects. Their attention to clinical detail and examination layout is greatly appreciated. A number of other medical students deserve our thanks for their helpful comments and suggestions (especially Richard McCrory) – many of which have been incorporated into this second edition.

The most important thank-you goes to many people who may never know of our gratitude. A group of people who, during times of trouble in unfamiliar environments, spare their time, patience and good nature – the patients.

Ian Bickle
Paul Hamilton

Clinical skills are the basis on which medical practice operates and despite technological advance are still the foundation of patient-based medicine. This book details the key examinations especially relevant to the medical student. All chapters refer to examination of adult patients. Techniques are explained in an easy-to-follow format, which, while being ideal for the newcomer to clinical examination, will also serve as a ready reference and revision guide for more senior students. The book does not aim to be extensive in covering all clinical examinations; nor does it detail every possible aspect of each specific examination – it is a practical guide to **essential** clinical skills. It contains what we term 'desert island' clinical skills – skills that, if you landed on a desert island, you could continue to practise.

The format is designed to be suitable for all students and combines practicality with foundation knowledge in examining systems of the body. This book includes major systems examinations, such as cardiovascular and respiratory, along with other regularly performed and important examinations of more isolated parts of the body, like the breast and thyroid gland.

You will also see the use of the VITAL POINT sign, which emphasises essential parts of the examination, which in some cases can be easily missed – not least with the nerves of an examination situation.

You should think about any clinical examination you carry out in the context of what we call the 'golden triangle':

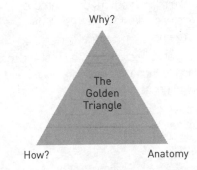

- Why the procedure is being carried out
- How to do the procedure
- Applying anatomical knowledge.

This triangle permits the application of knowledge and common sense in carrying out a useful rather than an idealistic but impractical examination.

Even in the days of early patient contact, a difficulty for most students is approaching patients with the confidence to carry out an examination. Although examining real patients with real pathology is the most fruitful, it is often valuable to practise routines on a willing friend or family member, until they become second nature.

You will notice that experienced clinicians can tailor a particular examination to the requirements of the patient. You should therefore use this booklet to provide you with a framework to fall back on. A methodical approach is needed that is flexible enough to undertake specific components as examination or hospital circumstances dictate.

Don't rely on examinations on their own! It is important to remember that the clinical examination is no substitute for a quality history, which can provide over 70% of all the information on which a diagnosis is based. For this reason a chapter is included detailing how to document a medical case, including the core questions for each system. You should carry out all examinations with the history you have elicited in mind – this will confirm or clarify your suspicions and detect additional or incidental findings. The history should be taken first where possible.

We hope that you will find this book both useful and enjoyable.

You will note that there have been three major additions in the second edition of this text:

• Standardised approach to major systems examinations: This incorporates the 'ICE' approach (introduction, consent and exposure). We hope that this will offer a familiar approach to begin each examination.

• An 'examination skeleton' completing each chapter: This will provide a rapid reference point for each system in the run-up to important medical school exams.

• Inclusion of a section on practical procedures: This will be of most relevance to those in the senior years, and will ease the transition from student to house officer.

Ian Bickle
Paul Hamilton

There are a number of simple, yet fundamental, points that need to be borne in mind when you are formally examining any patient. For ease of memory, work through the 'ICE' system when you begin any examination. If you are being observed and assessed, this will at least get you started, and will buy you some time to calm your nerves and gather your thoughts.

ICE system

- **I**ntroduce yourself. You should state your name and status (eg 'Hello. My name is Joe Bloggs, and I am a first-year medical student.') Shaking a patient's hand at this stage helps to build up a rapport.
- **C**onsent the patient for the examination (eg 'May I examine your hands please?').
- **E**xpose the necessary parts of the body and position the patient as necessary for the particular system or part being examined. Remember the patient's dignity, and provide a blanket or sheet to temporarily cover the patient if appropriate.

Some other pointers to keep at the back of your mind include:

- Always try to look professional, eg with regard to style of hair and clothing.
- Male students should be accompanied by a female chaperone when examining female patients.
- Ensure the patient is as comfortable as possible, in what is an unfamiliar environment.
- Examine from the right side except when this is not feasible.
- Ask if the body part to be examined is painful **before** touching it.
- If you are aware that a test is uncomfortable, or if you need the patient to be relaxed, employ distraction tactics, eg chat to the patient about something pleasant.
- Always pay attention to hygiene, eg washing hands thoroughly before and after examining a patient, and wearing gloves when necessary.
- Have short fingernails – long nails make percussion and palpation harder for you, and unpleasant for the patient.
- Always examine and compare similar structures on both sides of the body, even if you know only one side is abnormal.
- Warm your hands or any other object (eg stethoscope, tuning fork) that you are about to place on the patient's skin.
- When using a stethoscope, tap on the diaphragm to check it is not switched onto the bell.

- When measuring, ensure that the measurement is accurately reproducible by recording the distance from a fixed bony landmark.
- Listen to what the patient says, and respect their opinions at all times.
- Thank the patient at the end of an examination.

Medical records serve several functions.

A 'working document'

The recorded case history is a document recorded at the time of admission and the subsequent period of days, weeks or months of the patient's stay. It is used to record actual findings, results of tests, plans for future investigation, information received from relatives, healthcare workers and other interested parties and also how, why and when decisions were made regarding treatment options or changes to therapy.

A permanent record of a clinical event

The recording then serves as a permanent record of an event in time that can be rediscovered and assessed. This is of use during outpatient follow up.

A reference document for other staff

Patients admitted to hospital meet a variety of clinical staff, and a team of junior doctors often undertakes their medical management. The medical record is central to providing information that can be shared by all the medical staff involved. Provided records are updated and accurate, they facilitate continuity of care for the patient and allows staff to quickly become familiar with events which may have happened of which they were not aware.

A historical record of past events

Some illnesses evolve over a period of weeks, months or even years. Occasionally it is only by reviewing past medical records of isolated acute events that one can appreciate how an illness is evolving and realise the underlying diagnosis.

A legal document

Unfortunately this is becoming more and more important. Patients rightly expect the best clinical care from the medical profession. Sometimes patients or their relatives feel that the care and attention that was given was less than they needed, frankly poor or inappropriate. In such cases legal action may be taken and the medical records are always used to judge what actually happened. Also, for patients involved in road traffic accidents, industrial injury or exposed to hazards at work, legal action may ensue and medical information is required. Past medical records are an extremely important source of this information. For these reasons a medical record must comply with the requirements of a legal document.

Requirements of a legal document

- It must be clear who the records refer to – all documents must display the patient's name, date of birth and hospital number.
- Every entry in the records must be dated and signed. The author of the record must be identifiable. Therefore, you should always print name and designation, eg 'Senior House Officer', 'Medical Student'.
- Any changes in records should be signed and dated.
- No record should be falsified.
- No records should be deleted or removed unless a proper explanation is recorded, signed and dated by the individual responsible for the alteration.
- Medical records must be kept securely and available for inspection by the patient and their legal representatives if required.

As your clinical contact begins, you will no doubt be asked to write and present cases. This is an important technique to learn as it will not only help you study a variety of diseases, but it will stand you in good stead for clerking-in patients as a junior doctor. This chapter details the components of a comprehensive medical history and case report, and describes the rationale behind this approach. Two case reports (one medical and one surgical) have been included as examples. In addition an 'authentic' documented case is included.

All case reports should be tailored to the particular patient and their medical problem. For instance, a detailed social history is usually mandatory for any elderly patient, whereas some details may be omitted for a younger patient. If a patient presents with knee pain, you should document the knee and hip examinations in detail. In other cases, documentation of a GALS screen (gait, arms, legs, spine) may be more appropriate.

The components of a case report

- Basic patient details
- Presenting complaints
- History of presenting complaints
- Past medical history
- Drug history
- Family history
- Social and personal history
- Review of systems
- Physical examination

Basic patient details

Start with basic demographic details: name, age, date of birth, occupation, marital status, date of admission to hospital, consultant, location, hospital number and the date of your examination. These details are necessary, and asking for them allows you to gently ease the patient into questioning.

Keep patients' details confidential by using initials.

Presenting complaints

Ask the patient why they came to hospital. List each symptom in chronological order, along with its duration. Use the patient's words if possible.

History of presenting complaints

The history of presenting complaints should be written in a flowing commentary style in concise paragraphs.

Start with when the patient last felt well – this gives a starting point for the current illness.

Next, work your way through the symptoms listed in the 'Presenting complaints' section. Each symptom should be explored in detail. In particular, you should note how the symptoms have changed with time. For every given symptom, there are a variety of questions you should ask. You will learn these questions as your knowledge of diseases and exposure to patients increases. Pain is an extremely common symptom, and is used as an example below. The following headings will help your assessment:

- *Site*: Where is the pain?
- *Onset*: When did it come on? What were you doing? Did it come on suddenly?
- *Severity*: How severe is the pain on a scale from 1 to 10?
- *Character*: Describe the pain to me.
- *Radiation*: Does the pain go anywhere else?
- *Aggravating factors*: What makes the pain worse?
- *Relieving factors*: What makes the pain better?
- *Associated symptoms*: Are there any other symptoms with the pain, eg nausea?
- *Duration*: How long did the pain last?

When the patient has stopped volunteering useful information, you will need to start probing for more details. A good way to do this is to ask questions relating to the body systems that may be causing the patient's symptoms (see pages xviii and xix). For example, if the patient complains of chest pain, ask all the questions relating to the cardiovascular and respiratory systems.

At all times, when taking a history, you should be attempting to think of a diagnosis that may explain the patient's condition. At this stage in your patient assessment, there may be several diseases that could explain their symptoms. You should now ask questions directed at these differential diagnoses, with the aim of narrowing down your list of possibilities. In the chest pain example, you could ask whether the patient had been undertaking any unusual physical activity (since the pain may be due to muscular strain) and whether the patient has any major risk factors for ischaemic heart disease or pulmonary embolism.

Past medical history

Ask the patient about long-standing medical conditions, along with their date of diagnosis. Document any hospital admissions in chronological order.

Ask every patient specifically whether there is any history of: ischaemic heart disease, myocardial infarction, cerebrovascular disease, rheumatic fever, diabetes mellitus, hypertension, asthma, chronic obstructive airways disease, tuberculosis, jaundice and epilepsy.

Drug history

This has five major components.

> **Components of a drug history**
> - Current medication list
> - Allergy status
> - Alcohol consumption
> - Smoking
> - Recreational drug use

Current medication list

Accuracy and completeness are paramount in recording what medications a patient receives. Many patients carry a list of medications on their person. It is often worth asking to see this. This section should include all current medications, including over-the-counter preparations and alternative therapies. Any significant drugs used in the past such as cytotoxic agents, immunosuppressants and steroids should be noted. Record the drug name, dose, frequency of administration, route of administration and indications.

With the odd exception, medications should be written in their generic form. CAPITAL LETTERS should be used for clarity. For example, document OMEPRAZOLE rather than LOSEC®. Those preparations that include more than one drug or that are special formulations (such as slow- or modified-release) may need the proprietary (manufacturer's) name to be noted. For example, Adalat® SR is acceptable for the slow-release preparation of nifedipine. Medications administered in microgram doses, for example digoxin, should have the units written in full (ie write 125 micrograms, not 125 mcg). Never use a 'trailing zero' as it can easily result in an tenfold overdose (eg 2.0 mg could easily be mistaken for 20 mg). For drugs given by the frequency PRN (as required), a minimal time interval and/or maximum dose over 24 hours should be recorded.

When recording medications for children it is essential that the weight of the child (in kilograms) is recorded clearly. You should also specify the strength of any liquid preparations used.

Allergy status

Record if the patient has any drug allergies. If there are none, it is convention to write 'NKDA' (no known drug allergies). Ask specifically whether or nor the patient is allergic to penicillin.

Alcohol consumption

The number of units of alcohol consumed per day, week or month should be recorded, together with the pattern of alcohol intake (eg drinks daily, or binges occasionally). One unit of alcohol is equivalent to half a pint of standard-strength beer, one standard glass of wine, or a 25-ml measure of spirits.

Smoking

Tobacco can be chewed, sniffed (snuff) or inhaled. The number of cigarettes smoked each day or the amount (in grams/ounces) of tobacco used should be recorded. You may get a more accurate value by asking the number of packets/pouches purchased each week as patients invariably underestimate if asked directly. Find out when they started smoking. If they are a non-smoker, ask if they ever did smoke and, if so, how much and for how long. These values should then be converted into 'pack years'.

> **One pack year is equivalent to smoking 20 cigarettes a day for one year.**

'Recreational' drug use

If there is any indication or suspicion, patients should be asked about drugs of abuse, eg cannabis, narcotics, solvents. If these drugs have been used, it is vital to enquire about intravenous drug use and whether or not hypodermic needles have been shared with other users.

Family history

This section is to establish if there are any hereditary diseases in the patient's family. Details of the past or present ill health of parents, siblings, children (if any) and partner should be noted. The ages at which relatives developed ill health, as well as how and when relatives died should be recorded. You may find it useful to construct a family tree, especially if there is a strong family history.

Social and personal history

This is a vital section for the holistic approach to patient care. This aims to ascertain an insight into a patient's home environment and lifestyle. This is especially important for discharge purposes and for enrolling the help of other members of the healthcare team.

The following essential details should be recorded, where appropriate:

- Activities of daily living (transfer, dressing, washing, feeding)
- Location of bedroom and bathroom (eg upstairs or downstairs)
- House type (especially the number of flights of stairs) and any modifications (eg occupational therapy aids)
- Outside help (eg meals on wheels, district nurse)
- Family dynamics (who is at home, any dependants)
- Leisure activities and pets
- Recent foreign travel
- Level of education
- Financial status (especially any benefits received)
- Previous occupation(s) and description of work involved
- Exposure to potentially harmful materials (eg asbestos).

Review of systems

In order that you do not miss any important symptoms, a review of all body systems should be performed using directed questioning. There is no need to repeat the questions asked in the history of the presenting complaint. A thorough systems review is an essential part of any case history, since patients may fail to mention a vital symptom because they feel it is not relevant.

For any given system, there are a multitude of potential questions that could be asked. For practical purposes, a core set of questions should be asked of all patients for screening purposes. **These are asterisked in the box overleaf**. Further symptoms can be enquired about, should a particular system require in-depth exploration.

You might want to keep a copy of these questions in your white coat, especially to begin with, in order to become proficient in asking them.

Core questions for screening

General symptoms
- Weight change*
- Night sweats*
- Energy levels*

Cardiorespiratory systems
- Chest pain*
- Dyspnoea* (shortness of breath)
- Orthopnoea* (shortness of breath on lying flat)
- Paroxysmal nocturnal dyspnoea* (waking from sleep with dyspnoea)
- Cough*
- Sputum (quality, consistency, colour)*
- Haemoptysis* (coughing up blood)
- Wheezing*
- Ankle swelling*
- Palpitations*
- Syncope* (fainting)
- Intermittent claudication (pain in the calf/thigh/buttock on walking)

Alimentary system
- Nausea*
- Dysphagia* (difficulty swallowing)
- Vomiting*
- Haematemesis* (vomiting blood)
- Abdominal pain*
- Bowel habit* (diarrhoea or constipation)
- Rectal bleeding*
- Melaena* (foul-smelling, black, tarry stools)
- Appetite
- Thirst
- Mouth ulcers
- Heartburn
- Tenesmus (feeling the need to defecate even if rectum is empty)
- Colour of stools
- Mucus per rectum
- Steatorrhoea (whitish stools that are difficult to flush due to high fat content)

Nervous system
- Headaches*
- Vision*
- Blackouts*
- Fits*
- Dizziness*
- Loss of power*
- Sensory changes, including paraesthesia* (pins and needles)
- Mood
- Memory
- Vertigo (sensation that the surroundings are moving)
- Tinnitus (ringing in the ears)
- Balance
- Incontinence
- Speech disturbances
- Hearing
- Sleeping

Genitourinary system
- Hesitancy* (difficulty starting to pass urine)
- Altered stream* (eg poor flow)
- Dribbling*
- Dysuria* (burning sensation on passing urine)
- Frequency* (passing urine more than normal)
- Nocturia* (the need to pass urine when sleeping)
- Urgency* (a sudden unexpected desire to pass urine)
- Haematuria* (blood in the urine)

If relevant, in female patients
- Last menstrual period
- Regularity of period
- Length of period/cycle
- Heaviness of period
- Age at menarche (first menstrual cycle)
- Age at menopause
- Number of pregnancies

Locomotor
- Joint pain*
- Joint swelling*
- Joint stiffness*

Skin
- Itch*
- Rash*

> **Often the patient will not be able to remember some or all of their medical history. Don't forget that there are plenty of alternative sources if need be: family, friends, neighbours, old medial notes, family doctor and institutional sources (eg nursing home, school).**

Physical examination

General examination

Always record the following:

- General appearance, eg looks well; obviously in pain; cachectic elderly lady
- Temperature
- The presence or absence of 'JACCOL':
    - jaundice
    - anaemia of palmar creases and conjunctivae
    - cyanosis
    - clubbing (finger or toe)
    - oedema
    - lymphadenopathy
- The state of the mouth and throat, eg tongue moist and not coated; throat not injected
- The presence or absence of a goitre

Systems examinations

> **The system most related to the presenting complaint should be documented first.**

Thereafter the order does not really matter, although one general convention is: cardiovascular, respiratory, alimentary, nervous, and musculoskeletal.

The fundamentals of each system should be recorded, including the key negative findings. One of the best ways to see how to do this is to look at some well-recorded notes on a general medicine/surgery ward to get a feel for how it is done.

Summary

Summarise in one short paragraph the main points of note from the history and examination.

....
A good summary is a vital part of any case history, and should never be omitted.
....

Problem list

List, in order of priority, the problems that should be addressed in the management of the patient.

Differential diagnosis

A sensible range of possibilities should be considered, perhaps with some comment justifying why a particular disease has been included. The diseases should be arranged with the most likely coming first.

Investigations

Include a description of the investigations that should be performed, along with relevant results. Always start with simple investigations. Further tests may be requested based on the results of preliminary findings.

Definitive diagnosis

A statement of the most likely disease process, based on the history, physical examination, and investigations.

Management

Details of how the patient should be managed, both in the acute setting, and in the long term.

Commentary

This is included for academic purposes only (ie not found in 'real' patients' notes). The expectation of content for the commentary varies considerably between clinicians, and it is a good idea to find out what is expected in this section before it is written. Generally, one aspect of the case is chosen and explored in detail, with reference to the medical literature.

V Remember to date, sign and print your position/rank with all medical notes.

V If you have cited other authors' work in your commentary, remember to reference it correctly.

Example of a medical case report

Name:	Mrs I B
Age:	68 years
DOB:	22/09/1936
Occupation:	Retired civil servant
Marital status:	Married
Location:	Acute Admissions Ward
Hospital number:	XYZ-15978
Date of admission:	10/11/2004
Consultant:	Dr Bird
Examined on:	10/11/2004

Presenting complaints

- Epigastric discomfort – 1 month
- Lethargy – 3 weeks
- Shortness of breath – 10 days
- Palpitations – 1 day.

History of presenting complaints

Last felt perfectly well 1 month ago with background history of rheumatoid disease for 20 years.

Epigastric discomfort started 1 month ago. No previous problems with indigestion. Dull ache, no special relationship with eating. No radiation. Mild nausea only. No haematemesis. Stools on the darker side of late. No diarrhoea or constipation. No rectal bleeding. On NSAIDs.

Tired for past 3 weeks. Unable to carry out normal ADLs, and has been confined to the house for the past week. Increasingly tired over this period. This is despite regular sleep. Progressive shortness of breath. No previous problems of this nature. No respiratory history. Previous exercise tolerance on flat unlimited (more restricted by her arthritis). Now exercise tolerance of 30 yards. No associated chest pain. No cough, sputum, haemoptysis or wheeze. No ankle swelling, orthopnoea or paroxysmal nocturnal dyspnoea.

Her admission to hospital was confounded with the development of palpitations at rest 1 day ago. Felt dizzy, but did not pass out. Self-resolved in the ambulance to hospital, but since recurred in the Emergency Department.

Previous medical history

- 1984: rheumatoid disease
- 1987: arthrodesis of wrist (left)
- 1988: hypertension
- 1990: angina (mild). Last angina episode 6 months ago
- 1993: hypothyroidism
- 1996: phacoemulsification for cataract (right)
- 2000: total hip replacement (right)
- 2001: osteoporosis
- No history of myocardial infarction, rheumatic fever, diabetes mellitus, asthma, chronic obstructive airways disease, tuberculosis, jaundice or epilepsy.

Drug history

ASPIRIN ENTERIC COATED	75 mg	OD	PO	for secondary prevention of coronary artery disease
THYROXINE	100 micrograms	OD	PO	for hypothyroidism
METHOTREXATE	15 mg	WEEKLY	PO	for rheumatoid arthritis
IBUPROFEN	200 mg	TID	PO	for joint pains
FOLIC ACID	5 mg	WEEKLY	PO	as on methotrexate
RISEDRONATE	35 mg	WEEKLY	PO	for osteoporosis
ADALAT RETARD	10 mg	OD	PO	for angina prophylaxis
BENDROFLUMET-HIAZIDE	2.5 mg	OD	PO	for hypertension

Other:

- ALLERGIC TO SALAZOPYRIN
- Previously on steroids for several years
- Lifelong non-smoker
- Teetotal.

Family history

- Mother: rheumatoid disease. Still alive
- Sister (younger): pernicious anaemia. Still alive
- Sister (older): hypothyroidism. Still alive
- Husband: stroke 3 years ago at age 66 years. Limited mobility
- Children: alive and well.

Social and personal history

- Lives in housing association bungalow
- Husband at home
- Handrails outside property and inside the home
- Home help daily
- Walks with a stick for security.

Review of systems

- General: as above; nil else
- Alimentary: see history of presenting complaints
- Cardiorespiratory: see history of presenting complaints
- Locomotor: increasing hand pains recently; pain fairly well controlled on current medication
- Skin: nil of note
- Genitourinary: nil of note
- Nervous: nil of note.

Physical examination

General

- Pale appearance. Temperature 36.1 °C. Pallor of palmar creases and conjunctivae
- Tissue-paper skin in keeping with previous steroid use
- No jaundice, cyanosis, clubbing, oedema or lymphadenopathy
- Tongue moist and not coated. Throat not injected
- No goitre.

Alimentary system

- Abdomen normal in shape; moves normally with respiration. Abdomen soft. Mild tenderness in epigastric region. No organomegaly. No clinical abdominal aortic aneurysm. Easily reducible para-umbilical hernia. Bowel sounds normal. No bruits.

- Perianal skin normal. No anal fissures. Perianal sensation intact. Anal tone normal. No masses palpable in rectum. Normal faeces on glove.

Cardiovascular system

- Pulse 110 beats per minute, regular, normal character, normal volume, normal vessel wall, symmetrical. BP 106/56 mmHg. JVP not visible. Apex beat 6th intercostal space, mid-clavicular line. No heaves or thrills. First and second heart sounds normal. No added sounds. Short systolic murmur heard in all areas. No carotid bruits. Peripheral pulses intact.

Respiratory system

- Breathing comfortably. Respiratory rate 19 breaths per minute. No tremor or asterixis. Kyphotic with a small anteroposterior chest wall diameter. Trachea central. Cricosternal distance normal. Chest expansion good and symmetrical. Percussion note resonant in all areas. Breath sounds of normal intensity. Fine bilateral basal inspiratory crepitations. Vocal fremitus normal. Oxygen saturation 90% on room air.

Cranial nerves

- I: taste and smell reported to be normal
- II: pupils equal and reactive to light and accommodation. Visual fields full
- III/IV/VI: full range of eye movements
- V: sensation and motor functions intact. Jaw jerk negative
- VII: intact
- VIII: whisper test normal
- IX, X: normal voice, cough and swallow. Uvula central. Gag reflex intact
- XI: normal
- XII: tongue normal. Motor function intact.

Peripheral nervous system

- No tremor, muscle wasting, hypertrophy, asymmetry or abnormal posture. No fasciculation
- No pronator drift
- Upper limbs:
  - Tone normal
  - Power 5/5 in all muscle groups
  - Co-ordination normal. No dysdiadochokinesia
  - Reflexes normal
  - Sensation of light touch and pain intact in all dermatomes

- Lower limbs:
  - Tone normal
  - Power 5/5 in all muscle groups
  - Co-ordination normal
  - Reflexes normal. Plantar reflexes down-going
  - Sensation of light touch and pain intact in all dermatomes
  - Gait normal. Romberg's test negative.

GALS screen

- *Gait:* normal with a rapid turn
- *Spine:* thoracic kyphosis. No lumbar lordosis or scoliosis. The spine was not tender. Lumbar spine flexion was normal. Lateral flexion of the cervical spine was normal. There was no tenderness in the supraspinatus muscles
- *Arms:* shoulder and elbow movements were slightly painful. Symmetrical deforming arthritis of both hands. Hand grips were reduced. Mild pain upon squeezing laterally across the metacarpal-phalangeal (MCP) joints on either side. A single nodule was present over the extensor aspect of the right elbow
- *Legs:* internal rotation of the left hip was reduced. Knee flexion was normal, although crepitus was present. There was an obvious right knee effusion. There was no pain upon squeezing laterally across the metatarsal-phalangeal (MTP) joints on either side. There were some calluses on both feet.

Summary

A 68-year-old lady with 20-year history of rheumatoid disease on methotrexate and a NSAID. Multiple medical co-morbidities. Short history of epigastric discomfort and lethargy, accompanied more recently by shortness of breath and palpitations. On examination, pale, epigastric discomfort, and short systolic murmur. A right knee effusion is also noted.

Problem list

- Epigastric discomfort
- Shortness of breath
- Palpitations
- Heart murmur
- Right knee effusion
- Poor functional capacity.

Differential diagnosis

- NSAID-induced gastric bleed resulting in anaemia
- Poorly controlled thyroid disease
- Active rheumatoid disease
- Gastroduodenal ulcer
- Pernicious anaemia.

Investigations

Blood tests

A full blood picture is necessary since the patient is probably anaemic. The platelet count and white cell count could be reduced as an adverse effect of her methotrexate therapy. Liver function may also be impaired with this medication. ESR and CRP would be raised in active rheumatoid disease. A urea and electrolytes profile is essential to ascertain baseline renal function. This may affect the choice of any drug given to this patient.

Hb	6.8 g/dl	ESR	20 mm/h
WCC	5.46×10^9/litre	Platelets	334×10^9/litre
RCC	3.5×10^{12}/litre	Neutrophils	5.20×10^9/litre
HCT	0.32 l/litre	Lymphocytes	1.42×10^9/litre
MCV	70 fl	Monocytes	0.76×10^9/litre
MCH	25 pg	Eosinophils	0.13×10^9/litre
MCHC	25 g/dl	Basophils	0.05×10^9/litre
RDW	12.4%		
Sodium	134 mmol/litre	Alkaline phosphatase (ALP)	52 IU/litre
Potassium	3.8 mmol/litre	AST	28 IU/litre
Chloride	95 mmol/litre	ALT	22 IU/litre
Carbon dioxide	26 mmHg	γ-GT	30 IU/litre
Urea	6.3 mmol/litre	Albumin	36 g/litre
Glucose	4.5 mmol/litre	Calcium	2.23 mmol/litre
Creatinine	65 μmol/litre	Phosphate	0.95 mmol/litre
Total protein	65 g/litre	CRP	6 mg/litre
Total bilirubin	5 μmol/litre		

These tests reveal a microcytic hypochromic anaemia. All other tests are essentially normal.

Further blood tests which might prove useful include: iron studies; gastric parietal cell antibodies; intrinsic factor antibodies; coeliac disease screen; and thyroid function tests.

Chest X-ray

This would give a visual confirmation of the cardiomegaly detected on clinical examination. It may also give an explanation for the shortness of breath and the crepitations heard on examination. One might expect to see the interstitial shadowing of pulmonary fibrosis which may be related to rheumatoid disease itself or a side-effect of methotrexate therapy. Further imaging with high-resolution CT scanning may be indicated.

This revealed moderate cardiomegaly. Reticulonodular shadowing was present bibasally. The appearance was consistent with pulmonary fibrosis.

ECG

This is necessary because of the patient's tachycardia, epigastric discomfort and hypertension.

Heart rate was 105 beats per minute, sinus tachycardia. Normal axis. Normal QRS complexes. Meets the voltage criteria for left ventricular hypertrophy. No acute ST-segment or T-wave changes.

Pulmonary function tests

This would be necessary to investigate the possibility of pulmonary fibrosis, especially given the history of rheumatoid disease, the clinical findings and the chest X-ray appearance.

This revealed a restrictive pattern, in keeping with pulmonary fibrosis.

Oesophagogastroduodenoscopy (OGD)

This is to investigate the strong possibility that the patient's epigastric discomfort and anaemia may be due to a lesion in the upper gastrointestinal tract.

This revealed a 1.5 cm diameter ulcer in the posterior wall of the duodenum. A biopsy was taken.

The CLO test for *H.Pylori* was negative.

Multidisciplinary assessment

A full assessment by a physiotherapist and an occupational therapist would be beneficial in this patient.

Definitive diagnosis

NSAID-induced duodenal ulcer with resulting anaemia. Pulmonary fibrosis, most likely due to rheumatoid disease, was also detected.

Management

The NSAID should be discontinued, and replaced with simple analgesics. A proton pump inhibitor has been commenced. The patient should be transfused with 2 units of packed red cells initially, since she is symptomatic from her anaemia, especially in view of her IHD history. Repeat OGD has been arranged as an outpatient for 2 months' time.

Further attention should be given to the pulmonary fibrosis once the anaemia has been corrected. This is because the fibrosis is likely to have been a long-standing problem. Referral to a respiratory physician would be appropriate.

Example of a surgical case report

Name:	Mrs A B
Age:	72 years
DOB:	28/03/1932
Occupation:	Retired shop assistant
Marital status:	Widowed
Location:	Acute Admissions Ward
Hospital number:	ABC-15818
Date of admission:	10/06/2004
Consultant:	Mr Jones
Examined on:	12/06/2004

Presenting complaints

* Diarrhoea – 1 month.
* Rectal bleeding – 2 days.

History of presenting complaints

The patient last felt well several months ago.

Mrs B has been troubled with constipation for years, but in the last month has had diarrhoea, ie passing loose stools more often than usual, up to three times per day.

Two days ago, she noticed bleeding per rectum. She reports some bright red blood on the toilet paper. Additionally, there was blood mixed with the stools. She passed around half a cupful of blood on this occasion. She has passed a bowel motion on three further occasions since then, and on each occasion there has been some bleeding. The patient attributed the bleeding to haemorrhoids, which her general practitioner had diagnosed several years previously. The stools were not dark in colour, and the smell was no more offensive than usual.

Appetite has not been as good as previously in recent months. She has lost several pounds in weight over a 3-month period. There has been no nausea or vomiting. Thirst is normal. There is no reported mouth ulcers, dysphagia, vomiting or haematemesis. The patient reports some mild epigastric pain from time to time. There is no reported heartburn, indigestion, flatulence, tenesmus or steatorrhoea.

She had not been in contact with anyone else with diarrhoea recently, and had not been eating any unusual foods. There is no personal or family history of inflammatory bowel disease, bowel neoplasia or polyps. There has been no foreign travel.

Previous medical history

- As a child: appendicectomy
- 1995: diagnosed with hypertension
- 2002: stroke affecting the right side of the body; good recovery with no residual weakness
- No history of ischaemic heart disease, myocardial infarction, rheumatic fever, diabetes mellitus, asthma, chronic obstructive airways disease, tuberculosis, jaundice or epilepsy.

Drug history

ASPIRIN ENTERIC COATED	75 mg	OD	PO	for secondary prevention of cerebrovascular disease
BENDROFLUMETHIAZIDE	2.5 mg	OD	PO	for hypertension

Other:

- NKDA
- Lifelong non-smoker
- No alcohol.

Family history

- Father: died aged 76 years from myocardial infarction
- Mother: died aged 92 years from stroke
- Sister: alive, aged 84 years – hypertension
- Husband: died 10 years ago, aged 65 years– myocardial infarction
- Children: alive and well.

Social and personal history

- Lives alone in a pensioner's bungalow. Handrails fitted in the bathroom.
- Able to perform all activities of daily living unassisted
- Two daughters call in on a daily basis. No home helps
- Retired shop assistant.

Review of systems

- General: generally feeling tired, with poor energy in recent months
- Alimentary: see history of presenting complaints
- Cardiorespiratory: mild bilateral ankle swelling; nil else
- Locomotor: mild pain in both knees on walking long distances; nil else

- Skin: nil of note
- Genitourinary: nil of note
- Nervous: nil of note.

Physical examination

General

- Frail elderly lady. Temperature 36.2 °C. Mild bilateral pitting ankle oedema
- No jaundice, anaemia, cyanosis, clubbing or lymphadenopathy
- Tongue moist and not coated. Throat not injected
- No goitre.

Alimentary system

- Abdomen normal in shape; moves normally with respiration. Striae albicans. Hands normal
- Soft and non-tender. 5 x 5 cm hard, craggy, non-tender, mobile mass palpable in left lumbar region. No organomegaly. No clinical abdominal aortic aneurysm. Bowel sounds normal. No bruits
- Two small haemorrhoids visible perianally. No anal fissures. Perianal sensation intact. Anal tone normal. No masses palpable in rectum. Small amount of altered blood on glove.

Cardiovascular system

- Pulse 84 beats per minute, regular, normal character, normal volume, normal vessel wall, and symmetrical. BP 186/96 mmHg. JVP at 3 cm; normal character. Apex beat in 6th intercostal space, anterior axillary line. No heaves or thrills. Heart sounds I and II normal. No added sounds. No murmurs. Left-sided carotid bruit. Peripheral pulses intact.

Respiratory system

- Breathing comfortably. Respiratory rate 15 breaths per minute. No tremor or asterixis. No chest wall abnormalities. Trachea central. Cricosternal distance normal. Chest expansion good and symmetrical. Percussion note resonant in all areas. Breath sounds vesicular with no adventitious sounds. Vocal fremitus normal. Oxygen saturation 96% on room air.

Cranial nerves

- I: taste and smell reported to be normal
- II: pupils equal and reactive to light and accommodation. Visual fields full
- III, IV, VI: full range of eye movements
- V: sensation and motor functions intact. Jaw jerk negative
- VII: intact

- VIII: whisper test normal
- IX, X: normal voice, cough and swallow. Uvula central. Gag reflex intact
- XI: normal
- XII: tongue normal. Motor function intact.

Peripheral nervous system

- No tremor, muscle wasting, hypertrophy, asymmetry or abnormal posture. No fasciculation
- No pronator drift
- Upper limbs:
  - tone normal
  - power 5/5 in all muscle groups
  - co-ordination normal. No dysdiadochokinesia
  - reflexes normal
  - sensation of light touch and pain intact in all dermatomes
- Lower limbs:
  - tone normal
  - power 5/5 in all muscle groups
  - co-ordination normal
  - reflexes normal. Plantar reflexes down-going
  - sensation of light touch and pain intact in all dermatomes
  - gait normal. Romberg's test negative.

GALS screen

- *Gait:* normal with a rapid turn
- *Spine:* no thoracic kyphosis, lumbar lordosis or scoliosis. Spine not tender. Lumbar spine flexion normal. Lateral flexion of the cervical spine normal. No tenderness in the supraspinatus muscles
- *Arms:* shoulder and elbow movements normal. Hand grips normal. No pain on squeezing laterally across the metacarpophalangeal (MCP) joints on either side .
- *Legs:* passive internal rotation of the hips normal. Knee flexion normal, and no crepitus. No pain on squeezing laterally across the metatarsalophalangeal (MTP) joints on either side. Some calluses on both feet.

Summary

A 72-year-old independent lady with a history of hypertension and stroke presents with a 2-day history of rectal bleeding and a 1-month history of altered bowel habit. A 5 x 5 cm, hard, mobile mass palpable in left lumbar region and haemorrhoids detected on clinical examination.

Problem list

- What is the cause of the rectal bleeding and altered bowel habit?
- Poorly controlled hypertension
- Left-sided carotid bruit.

Differential diagnosis

Large bowel neoplasia must be excluded as cause of this lady's symptoms. Other alternatives include: diverticular disease with palpable sigmoid colon, bowel polyps or inflammatory bowel disease. An infective cause for diarrhoea also remains a possibility, although an abdominal mass would not be a typical finding.

Investigations

Blood tests

A full blood picture is necessary since the patient may be anaemic owing to bleeding from a colonic neoplasm or polyp. White cell count, ESR and CRP may be raised with infective diarrhoea or diverticulitis. Liver function may be deranged if liver metastases are present. Urea and electrolytes profile is essential to ascertain baseline renal function. This may affect the choice of any drug given to this patient.

Hb	11.4 g/dl	ESR	25 mm/h
WCC	8.92 x 10⁹/litre	Platelets	334 x 10⁹/litre
RCC	4.94 x 10¹²/litre	Neutrophils	4.91 x 10⁹/litre
HCT	0.430 l/litre	Lymphocytes	2.58 x 10⁹/litre
MCV	87.0 fl	Monocytes	0.80 x 109/litre
MCH	29.1 pg	Eosinophils	0.63 x 10⁹/litre
MCHC	35.5 g/dl	Basophils	0.00 x 10⁹/litre
RDW	12.4%		
Sodium	138 mmol/litre	Alkaline phosphatase (ALP)	145 IU/litre
Potassium	4.3 mmol/litre	AST	23 IU/litre
Chloride	101 mmol/litre	ALT	20 IU/litre
Carbon dioxide	24 mmHg	γ-GT	42 IU/litre
Urea	6.1 mmol/litre	Albumin	36 g/litre
Glucose	5.6 mmol/litre	Calcium	2.34 mmol/litre
Creatinine	80 μmol/litre	Phosphate	1.03 mmol/litre
Total protein	71 g/litre	CRP	< 2 mg/litre
Total bilirubin	8 μmol/litre		

Stool culture

This is necessary to investigate the possibility of infective diarrhoea. It revealed no significant growth.

Chest X-ray

This could detect lung metastases from a colonic neoplasm, and would give a visual confirmation of the cardiomegaly detected on clinical examination. It revealed gross cardiomegaly. The lung fields were clear, and there was no evidence of pulmonary metastases.

ECG

This is necessary because of the patient's hypertension. ECG showed 82 beats per minute, normal sinus rhythm. Normal axis. Normal QRS complexes. Meets the voltage criteria for left ventricular hypertrophy. Strain pattern present. No acute ST-segment or T-wave changes.

Visualisation of the lower gastrointestinal tract

Definitive investigation in this patient's case would require visualisation of the large bowel. This could be done endoscopically, with flexible sigmoidoscopy in the first instance. Colonoscopy would be needed to visualise the entire colon. The bowel could alternatively be investigated radiologically with a double-contrast barium enema, although this would not allow biopsy of any suspicious lesion.

The patient underwent colonoscopy. This revealed a suspicious lesion in the distal descending colon. The rest of the large bowel and terminal ileum was visualised and was normal. Biopsy revealed colonic adenocarcinoma.

Further investigation

Further tests that could be carried out on this patient include abdominal imaging. An ultrasound scan, or ideally a CT scan, initially of the abdomen, should be carried out to stage the neoplastic disease.

If surgery is planned, the patient will need work-up for surgery. This will require:

- coagulation screen
- blood group and hold
- an echocardiogram to assess cardiac function
- possibly pulmonary function testing.

Definitive diagnosis

Adenocarcinoma of the descending colon.

Management

After assessment of fitness for surgery, this patient will undergo a left hemicolectomy, with resection of associated mesentery and regional lymph nodes. Consideration will be given as to whether a stoma will be fashioned, or whether an end-to-end bowel anastomosis will be carried out. A decision on any further therapy will be made following the clinicopathological conference.

Longer-term management of this patient should also address her poorly controlled hypertension and her carotid artery atherosclerosis (as evidenced by the carotid bruit).

The following pages contain an example of a 'real' medical case. This has been included to illustrate how the process of documenting a case is done in day to day medical practice. You will note the use of abbreviations and short-hand which are in common use. These should be avoided when preparing cases for formal assessment purposes.

ANYWHERE HOSPITAL

FORM C
CONTINUATION SHEET

NAME: HRS CHARLOTTE HAMILTON 12/04/39   HPN01010-14

DATE

27/11/04 Sho IAN BICKLE, 1715 HRS, WARD 5
          DR BIRDS TEAM

(65), Retired Postmistress (Married)

REF : Admission directed from clinic

PC: 1/ Abdominal discomfort   6 WEEKS
    2/ Low Energy   1 MONTH
    3/ Shortness of breath   5 DAYS
    4/ Palpitations   1 DAY

HPC: hard perfectly well 6 weeks ago

20 year history of Rheumatoid disease
On Methotrexate 15MG Weekly

Abdominal discomfort - epigastric
Nauseated at times. No Vomiting
No haematemesis. No strong relationship to food
Stools darker recently. ON NSAID ✓

Tired for 1 month. ADL more of a struggle. Disturbed sleep

Short of breath 100 yards. Previously unlimited.
No chronic chest disease. No sputum/cough.

This AM palpitations. Self resolving. No associated chest pain

(CONTINUED)

DATE

Past Medical History: Rheumatoid disease 1984

Pernicious Anaemia 1986

Hysterectomy 1991

Hypertension 1995

Hypothyroidism 1999

Right Wrist Arthrodesis 2002

Cataracts: Awaiting Surgery

No th of IHD / Rheumatic Fever / Epilepsy / Jaundice / Diabetes
Asthma / COPD / TB

Drug History: ALLERGIC TO DISTAMINE

Atenolol 50 MG OD Po

Folic Acid 5 MG WEEKLY (Fridays) Po

Methotrexate 15 MG WEEKLY Po

Celecoxib 200 MG OD Po

Tramadol SR 50 MG BD Po

Thyroxine 125 micrograms OD Po

Previously on steroids for long duration

Non - Smoker

C2 H5OH / wk = 2-4 units

Family Hx:

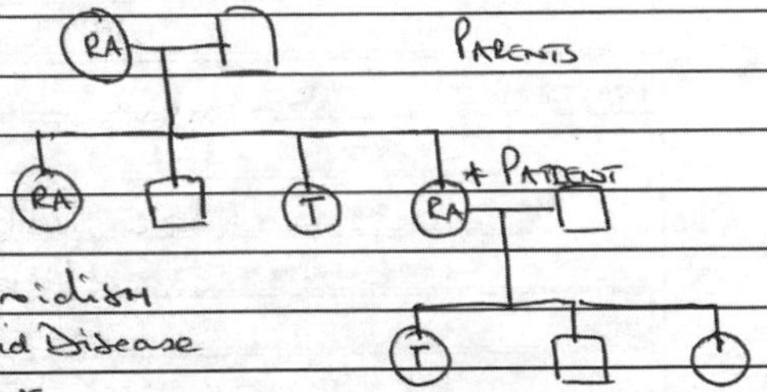

RA — [ ]   PARENTS

RA [ ]   (T) (RA) * PATIENT [ ]

T = Hypothyroidism
RA = Rheumatoid Disease

(T) [ ] ( )

ALL STILL ALIVE

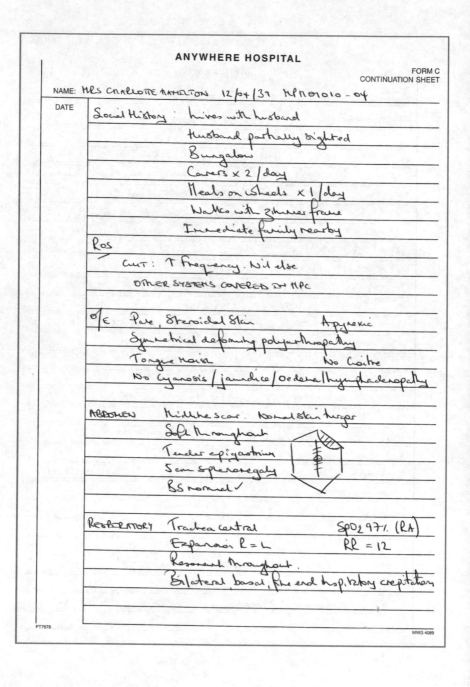

ANYWHERE HOSPITAL

FORM C
CONTINUATION SHEET

NAME: MRS CHARLOTTE HAMILTON   12/04/39   MHH01010-04

DATE

Social History : Lives with husband
Husband partially sighted
Bungalow
Carers x 2 / day
Meals on wheels x 1 / day
Walks with zimmer frame
Immediate family nearby

ROS

CVT: ↑ Frequency. Nil else

OTHER SYSTEMS COVERED IN HPC

O/E   Pale, Steroidal Skin   Apyrexic
Symmetrical deforming polyarthropathy
Tongue moist   No Goitre
No Cyanosis / jaundice / oedema / lymphadenopathy

ABDOMEN   Midline scar. Normal skin turgor
Soft throughout
Tender epigastrium
5cm splenomegaly
BS normal ✓

RESPIRATORY   Trachea central   SpO2 97% (RA)
Expansion R = L   RR = 12
Resonant throughout.
Bilateral basal, fine end inspiratory crepitations

PT7678

WWG 4089

(CONTINUED)

DATE

CARDIOVASCULAR :   Pulse 106, Regular, Good Volume

BP 108/48

JVP ⟷   No carotid bruit

HS I + II + Short Systolic murmur (all areas)

No peripheral oedema

CRANIAL NERVES

I ✓

II, III, IV, VI   PERLA. Full visual Fields. From. Fundi ⊖

V   MOTOR ✓   SENSORY ✓

VII ✓

VIII   WHISPER TEST NORMAL

IX, X   Gag intact, uvula central, cough ✓

XI, XII ✓

UPPER LIMB

		R	L	
TONE		(N)	(N)	
POWER		5/5	5/5	All Muscle Groups
COORDINATION		(N)	(N)	
REFLEXES	B	++	++	
	S	++	++	
	T	++	++	
SENSATION		Intact all modalities		

ANYWHERE HOSPITAL

FORM C
CONTINUATION SHEET

NAME: MRS CHARLOTTE HAMILTON 12/04/39 MRN 01010-04

DATE

LOWER LIMB

		R	L	
TONE		(N)	(N)	
POWER		5/5	5/5	ALL MUSCLE GROUPS
COORDINATION		(N)	(N)	
REFLEXES	K	++	++	
	A	++	++	
	PLANTARS	↓	↓	
SENSATION		Intact all modalities		

GALS SCREEN

Gait: Requires walking aid

Spine: Normal

Arms: Symmetrical deforming small joint polyarthropathy
MCP Squeeze tender bilaterally
Poor grip. Right wrist arthrodesis

Legs: Moderate Right knee effusion
↓ Internal rotation left hip

SUMMARY (65) 20 year history of Rheumatoid disease on
Methotrexate. Recent history of epigastric discomfort, low
energy, SOB and palpitations. On NSAID
O/E Tachycardic, systolic murmur, epigastric discomfort
and 5 cm splenomegaly. (R) knee effusion

(CONTINUED)

PROBLEM LIST

DATE

1/ Shortness of breath
2/ Palpitation
3/ Epigastric discomfort with dark stools
4/ Splenomegaly
5/ Right knee Effusion
6/ Heart murmur

LIKELY DIAGNOSIS: NSAID induced gastritis (→ Symptomatic anaemia)

DIFFERENTIAL DIAGNOSES: Peptic Ulcer
Pernicious anaemia (poorly controlled)
Hypothyroidism (poorly controlled)
Felty's Syndrome
Bacterial Endocarditis

MANAGEMENT

Investigation 1/ Bloods: FBP | U&E | LOAC | CRP | ESR | TFTs | B12 | FOLATE
IRON STUDIES / INTRINSIC FACTOR ANTIBODIES
X 3 BLOOD CULTURES

2/ Endoscopy: OGD ± biopsies

3/ ECG + Echo

4/ Imaging: Ultrasound Abdomen, ® knee x-ray

Treatment
1/ Discontinue NSAIDS. Replace with simple analgesia
2/ Commence Proton pump inhibitor
3/ Transfuse if Haemoglobin < 8 g/dl
4/ Aspirate ® knee effusion

J Pringle
(SHO)
BLEEP 1007

Presenting a clinical case is an exercise in efficient verbal communication. There are several reasons why medical students are asked to present cases:

- It is an excellent way of testing verbal communication skills.
- It represents a quick method of assessing history-taking and examination skills.
- Ultimately, it will prepare you for being a junior doctor, when an important part of the job involves discussing patients with senior staff.

It is important to sound confident when presenting, and to talk in a clear and coherent manner. Aim to include all essential information (as well as important negatives), but try to be concise and logical. Presentation of a case usually follows a conventional order which mimics a written case. An example case presentation is given below for guidance. This would be the verbal equivalent of the written surgical case report given on page xxxi.

Always remember confidentiality, and use initials where appropriate.

Try to make eye contact with the listener during any presentation.

Example of presenting a case history

'Mrs B is a 72-year-old widow who is a retired shop assistant. She was admitted on the 12th of June with a 2-day history of rectal bleeding and a 1-month history of diarrhoea. She last felt well several months ago. The patient would usually be constipated, but in the last month has been passing loose stools up to three times per day. The rectal bleeding consisted of noticing bright-red blood on the toilet paper, as well as blood in her stools. Around half a cup of blood was passed. Small amounts of bleeding are still occurring on defecation. Appetite is poor, and she has lost a small amount of weight. Mrs B reports having mild epigastric pain, but denies any further gastrointestinal symptoms. In particular, there is no tenesmus. She has had no contact with others with diarrhoea. There is no personal or family history of inflammatory bowel disease, bowel neoplasia or polyps.

Her past medical history includes hypertension. She had a stroke in 2002, but has no residual weakness. She is being treated with aspirin and bendroflumethiazide. She does not smoke or take alcohol. There is a strong family history of cardiovascular disease. She lives alone in a bungalow and manages well with minimal assistance.

Systematic questioning revealed poor energy recently, and mild ankle swelling.

On examination, Mrs B appeared frail. She was apyrexic and had mild bilateral pitting ankle oedema. There was no clinical jaundice or anaemia. Abdominal examination revealed a 5 x 5 cm, hard, craggy, non-tender, mobile mass in the left lumbar region. There was no organomegaly. Rectal examination revealed haemorrhoids and altered blood in the rectum. There were no rectal masses. Cardiovascular system examination revealed a blood pressure of 186/96 mmHg and a left carotid bruit. Other systems were unremarkable.

This lady's medical problems include: her rectal bleeding and altered bowel habit; her hypertension; and a left carotid bruit. The differential diagnosis includes bowel neoplasia, diverticular disease, bowel polyps, infective diarrhoea and inflammatory bowel disease.

This lady should be investigated initially with a full blood count, inflammatory markers, urea and electrolytes profile and liver function tests. Stool culture is also necessary. I would carry out an ECG and chest X-ray. Ultimately, this patient requires lower GI tract visualisation. Ideally this would involve colonoscopy, but barium enema with sigmoidoscopy would also be acceptable.'

SECTION 1
SYSTEMS-BASED EXAMINATIONS

ICE

- Introduce yourself.
- Consent the patient for the examination.
- Expose the necessary parts of the body and position the patient. Remove the shirt/blouse, and roll up trouser legs to expose the thorax and ankles respectively. Cover ladies with a blanket when not examining the heart. Position the back of the bed at 45° to the horizontal.

Examination

Inspection

From the end of the bed

- Look around the bed for clues, eg fluid restriction signs, GTN spray, diabetic biscuits.
- Scan the patient from head to toe, and note:
  - Does the patient look well or unwell?
  - Does the patient have any obvious conditions associated with cardiovascular disease, eg Down's syndrome?
  - Does the patient have any clues to cardiac disease that are immediately apparent, eg malar flush?
- What is the breathing pattern?
- Are the ankles obviously swollen?
- Is there a scar on the leg indicating previous bypass surgery?
- What is the patient's colour, eg pale, cyanosed, jaundiced, ruddy complexion?

Hands

Take the patient's hands in yours and look for:

- finger clubbing
- anaemia of palmar creases
- peripheral cyanosis
- evidence of smoking
- tendon xanthomata
- signs of infective endocarditis (splinter haemorrhages, Osler's nodes, Janeway lesions, petechiae).

Face

Scan the eyes and face and look for:

- xanthelasma
- corneal arcus
- malar flush.

Inspect the conjunctivae for anaemia, and look at the lips and tongue for central cyanosis.

Examine the radial pulse

Use two fingers. Press slightly harder with the distal finger (the one furthest away from the heart), thus 'amplifying' the pulse transmitted to the other finger.

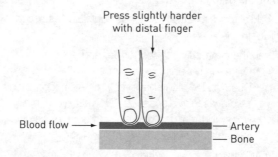

Note the following six features of the pulse:

- Rate (beats per minute)
- Rhythm (regular, regularly irregular, irregularly irregular)
- Character (eg normal, collapsing)
- Volume (low, normal, high)
- Vessel wall characteristics (normal, thickened)
- Symmetry (symmetrical, asymmetrical) – feel both radial pulses simultaneously to do this.

Test for a collapsing pulse:

- Feel for the radial pulse on one side. Keep your hands in the same position, and elevate the patient's arm above their head. Abnormal pulsation may indicate a collapsing pulse – a sign of aortic regurgitation.

Test for radiofemoral delay:

- Palpate the radial and femoral pulses on the same side, at the same time. A significant delay between the two is called 'radiofemoral delay', and is a sign of coarctation of the aorta.

Measure the blood pressure

- The patient should be as relaxed as possible, and should have been resting for some time before the measurement. Blood pressure is usually measured seated.

- Choose a suitably sized cuff, and wrap it securely around the patient's arm. Palpate the brachial artery in the antebrachial fossa, and adjust the cuff position so that it is in the correct position. (There is usually a mark on the cuff which should be lined up with the brachial artery.)

Place the sphygmomanometer at the level of the heart.

- Close the valve on the sphygmomanometer.

- Palpate the pulse at the radial artery, and inflate the cuff to about 30 mmHg over the level at which the pulse disappears.

- Auscultate over the brachial artery with the stethoscope diaphragm.

- Partly open the valve, so that the cuff pressure falls at a rate of about 2 mmHg per second.

- Note the pressure at which you begin to hear rhythmical noises. These noises are Korotkoff sounds, and the pressure when they start represents systolic blood pressure. Note the pressure at which the sounds disappear. This represents diastolic blood pressure. If the sounds do not disappear, the pressure at which they become muffled should be noted. The measurement should be repeated at least once.

- Compare the pressure with the patient sitting and after 2 minutes of standing. A systolic change of more than 20 mmHg between positions is indicative of postural hypotension.

Assess jugular venous pressure (JVP)

- Have the patient turn their head slightly to the left side.

- Ensure the area over the internal jugular vein is well illuminated (use a lamp).

- Look carefully for any pulsations.

- Verify that pulsations are not arterial (by checking for the JVP features listed in the box overleaf).

- The level of the JVP should be noted as in the diagram, by measuring the vertical height between the angle of Louis and the top of the venous column (normal < 3 cm).

- Check for hepatojugular reflux: While closely watching the patient's neck, gradually apply firm pressure over the liver, and hold for 4–5 seconds. A rise in the position of pulsation is indicative of a positive reflux. Ask the patient if there is any pain or tenderness before doing this, and tell the patient to breathe normally during the test.

Features of a JVP

- Pulsations cannot be palpated
- Can be easily occluded
- Fills from above
- Has at least two positive waveforms
- Varies with respiration, posture and hepatojugular reflux

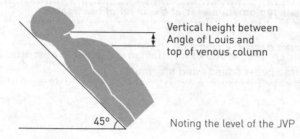

Vertical height between
Angle of Louis and
top of venous column

45°

Noting the level of the JVP

Praecordium (chest)

Inspection

Look for:

- scars: median sternotomy scars in the centre of the sternum (coronary artery bypass or aortic valve surgery), and lateral thoracotomy laterally on the chest (mitral valve surgery)
- pacemakers/implantable defibrillator devices
- abnormal pulsations
- a visible apex beat (see below).

Palpation

Palpate for:

- apex beat (the most lateral and inferior position in which the heart can be palpated). Note its position in anatomical terms, eg 5th intercostal space (ICS), mid-clavicular line
- heaves (forceful ventricular contractions)
- thrills (palpable murmurs).

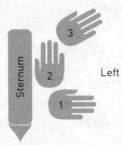

Right   Sternum   Left

Hand positions for palpating heaves and thrills. Numbers indicate the order in which the positions should be used

Auscultate the heart

Always palpate the carotid or subclavian pulse when auscultating, to help you time heart sounds and murmurs.

- During auscultation, listen for heart sounds (1, 2, 3 and 4), murmurs and any other abnormalities, eg clicks. Distinguish systolic from diastolic abnormalities by noting the relationship of the abnormality to the pulse. If the abnormality occurs when you feel a pulse, it is in systole. If it occurs when there is no pulse, it is in diastole.
- Listen in the mitral valve area with the stethoscope bell. Roll the patient onto their left side. Relocate the apex beat, and listen again at the apex beat and axilla with the bell. Listen specifically for the mid-diastolic murmur of mitral stenosis.
- Roll the patient onto their back again. Auscultate the four valve areas (see diagram below) with the stethoscope diaphragm.
- Ask the patient to lean forward off the bed, to exhale and hold their breath. Listen over the tricuspid and aortic areas. Listen specifically for the early diastolic murmur of aortic regurgitation.
- Ask the patient to hold their breath, and then auscultate over the carotid arteries for bruits.

Main areas for auscultation with diaphragm of stethoscope
1: Mitral area   apex beat
2: Tricuspid area   left 4th ICS
3: Pulmonary area   left 2nd ICS
4: Aortic area   right 2nd ICS

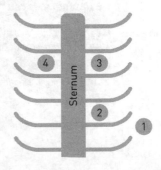

Examine the praecordium from behind

- Percuss the chest for dullness, which may indicate a pleural effusion.
- Listen over the lung bases for inspiratory crepitations, that are often present in left heart failure.
- Press over the sacrum to test for sacral oedema.
- Test for ankle oedema. Press on the anterior aspect of the ankle for up to 1 minute. Release your finger, and inspect for 'pitting'. This is common in right heart failure.

Thank the patient

Turn and face the examiner

State that you would like to complete the examination by:

1 Palpating the peripheral pulses:

- palpate the brachial (in the antebrachial fossa), femoral (in the groin), popliteal (in the popliteal fossa), posterior tibial (behind the medial malleolus at the ankle) and dorsalis pedis (on the top of the foot in line with the second toe) pulses

2 Assessing the abdomen:

- palpate the liver, which may be enlarged in right heart failure, or pulsatile in tricuspid regurgitation
- palpate the spleen, which may be enlarged in infective endocarditis
- palpate for an abdominal aortic aneurysm
- auscultate for bruits

3 Assessing the temperature chart

4 Performing fundoscopy (for hypertensive changes and signs of infective endocarditis)

5 Performing urinalysis.

Examiners' favourites

Q Name some cardiac causes of finger clubbing.

A Congenital cyanotic heart disease, infective endocarditis, atrial myxoma.

Q Why might the apex beat not be palpable on the left side?

A Obesity, excessive muscle bulk, hyperinflated lungs, dextrocardia, pericardial effusion.

Summary

ICE

▼

Inspect from the end of the bed

▼

Inspect the hands

▼

Inspect the face

▼

Examine the radial pulse

▼

Measure the blood pressure

▼

Assess the JVP

▼

Inspect the praecordium from the front

▼

Palpate the praecordium from the front

▼

Auscultate the heart from the front

▼

Examine the praecordium from behind the patient

▼

Test for ankle oedema

▼

Thank the patient

▼

Turn and face the examiner

ICE

- **I**ntroduce yourself.
- **C**onsent the patient for the examination.
- **E**xpose the necessary parts of the body and position the patient. Remove the shirt/blouse to expose the thorax. Cover ladies with a blanket when not examining the chest. Position the back of the bed at 45° to the horizontal.

Examination

Inspection

From the end of the bed

- Look around the bed for clues, eg peak-flow meters, inhalers, oxygen masks, sputum pots, non-invasive ventilation machine.
- Scan the patient from head to toe, and note:
  - Does the patient look well or unwell?
  - Does the patient have any obvious conditions, eg Cushing's syndrome?
  - Does the patient have any clues to respiratory disease that are immediately apparent, eg a chest drain?
  - What is their breathing pattern and are they using accessory muscles of respiration?
  - What is their respiratory rate?
  - Are they making any abnormal noises, eg wheeze, stridor?
  - What is the patient's colour, eg pale, cyanosed, jaundiced, ruddy complexion?

Hands

Take the patient's hands in yours and look for:

- finger clubbing
- anaemia of palmar creases
- peripheral cyanosis
- evidence of smoking

Test for tremor and carbon dioxide retention flap (asterixis):

- Ask the patient to put their arms straight out in front of them and fan their fingers apart. Look for a fine tremor (this may indicate use of a β_2-adrenoceptor agonist).
- Passively extend the wrists with the arms outstretched. Involuntary flexion may represent a CO_2 retention flap.

Face

- Scan the eyes and face and look for:
  - ptosis (drooping upper eyelid)
  - miosis (constricted pupil on one side)
  - enophthalmos (a sunken eye).

  These are three features of Horner's syndrome that may indicate an apical lung cancer.

- Inspect the conjunctivae for anaemia and chemosis (oedema, which may indicate carbon dioxide retention).
- Look at the lips and tongue for central cyanosis.

Examine the radial pulse

See the cardiovascular system examination.

Examine cervical and axillary lymph nodes

See the cervical lymph nodes and breast examinations.

Assess jugular venous pressure

See the cardiovascular system examination.

For the following four sections, perform all tests on the front of the chest.

Praecordium

Inspection

Look for:

- chest wall deformities, eg pectus excavatum/carinatum, kyphosis, scoliosis
- scars anteriorly or laterally
- overexpansion (inspect from the side).

Palpation

- Palpate the trachea to assess for deviation. Gently place the index and middle fingers on either side of the trachea in the suprasternal notch.

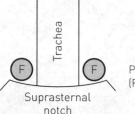

Palpation of the trachea
(F = position of finger)

- Palpate the cricosternal distance: finger-breadth distance between cricoid cartilage and suprasternal notch.
- Asses the amount and symmetry of chest expansion. Place your hands as shown in the diagram (the thumbs must be off the chest and meet in the midline). Ask the patient to take deep breaths in and out. Note how far your thumbs separate with each inspiration.

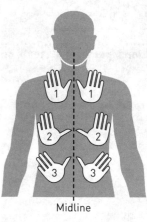

Position of hands for assessing chest expansion

- Palpate the left parasternal area for a right ventricular heave, by placing your finger tips in the intercostal spaces just to the left of the sternum. This may be felt in pulmonary hypertension.
- Palpate for the apex beat (see cardiovascular examination).
- Palpate for tactile fremitus. Rest the ulnar aspect of the hand on the chest wall, and ask the patient to say '99'. Note any abnormal vibrations. Do this at least six times – once in each of the hand positions on the above diagram. Always compare left and right sides.

Percussion

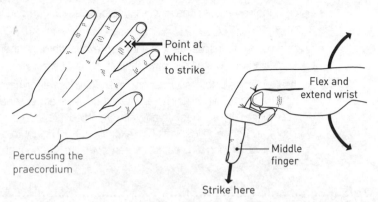

Point at which to strike

Percussing the praecordium

Flex and extend wrist

Middle finger

Strike here

- Percuss the praecordium by spreading out the fingers of one hand and resting the palm and fingers on the chest wall. Position your middle finger in an intercostal space. Strike the middle phalanx of this finger with the tip of the middle finger of the other hand. This technique needs lots of practice! (See diagram)
- Percuss the supraclavicular regions, the clavicles (tap each clavicle directly, ie don't tap your finger), the chest wall (in at least six positions to cover the entire lung fields) and the axillae.

Ⓥ Always compare left with right, by assessing both sides at each level.

- Determine whether the note is resonant (normal), hyper-resonant, dull or stony-dull.

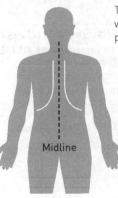

The curved lines indicate the 'path' which should be taken during percussion and auscultation

Midline

Auscultation (with diaphragm of stethoscope)

- Listen in the same positions in which you percussed, comparing sides at all times.
- Ask the patient to inspire deeply and then exhale (through the mouth) in each position of the stethoscope.
- Assess: whether breath sounds are vesicular (normal) or bronchial; the intensity of the breath sounds; and whether there are any adventitious (additional) breath sounds. If any abnormalities are heard, determine whether they occur on inspiration or expiration. If you want to experience the sound of bronchial breathing listen over the trachea of a healthy individual.

Remember patients may become dizzy if they are asked to inspire and expire deeply for prolonged periods.

> **Characteristics of breath sounds**
> - Intensity
> - Pitch
> - Ratio of inspiratory:expiratory phases
> - Presence/absence of pause between inspiration and expiration
> - Presence and timing of adventitious sounds: wheeze (rhonchi), crepitations (crackles)
> - Other sounds, eg pleural rub

- Assess vocal fremitus, by asking the patient to say '99' when you are auscultating. This is more reliable than tactile fremitus.

It is helpful to think of the anatomy of the lungs on percussion, palpation and auscultation to ensure that all lobes have been covered.

Go back and perform the previous four sections on the back of the chest.

Palpation from behind need only include assessment of chest expansion and tactile fremitus.

Thank the patient

Turn and face the examiner

State that you would like to complete the examination by:

- auscultating the heart (since cardiac and respiratory diseases are often linked)
- observing the temperature chart
- testing the peak expiratory flow rate.

Ensure that you ask to see any chest radiographs, lung function test results (spirometry and peak expiratory flow) and review the sputum pot contents.

Examiners' favourites

Q Name some respiratory causes of finger clubbing.

A Chronic suppurative lung disease, eg cystic fibrosis and bronchiectasis; lung cancer; mesothelioma.

Q What is central cyanosis?

A A bluish discoloration of the lips and tongue when the concentration of deoxyhaemoglobin in the blood exceeds 5 g/dl.

Summary

ICE
▼
Inspect from the end of the bed
▼
Inspect the hands
▼
Inspect the face
▼
Examine the radial pulse
▼
Examine the lymph nodes
▼
Assess the JVP
▼
Inspect the praecordium from the front
▼
Palpate the praecordium from the front
▼
Percuss the praecordium from the front
▼
Auscultate the praecordium from the front
▼
Inspect the praecordium from the back
▼
Palpate the praecordium from the back
▼
Percuss the praecordium from the back
▼
Auscultate the praecordium from the back
▼
Thank the patient
▼
Turn and face the examiner

> It is important to distinguish between examining the alimentary system (mouth to anus) and the abdomen. Examination of the abdomen is only a part of the full alimentary system examination.

ICE

- **I**ntroduce yourself.
- **C**onsent the patient for the examination.
- **E**xpose the necessary parts of the body and position the patient. Expose the abdomen from nipples to groins. Preserve the patient's dignity at all times and cover sensitive areas. Position the patient flat on the bed whenever possible, with the head on a single pillow. Arms and legs should be straight.

Examination

Inspection

From the end of the bed

- Look around the bed for clues, eg gluten-free biscuits, kidney dishes for vomiting, special dietary notices, 'nil by mouth' instructions.
- Scan the patient from head to toe, and note:
  - Does the patient look well or unwell?
  - Does the patient have any obvious conditions, eg systemic sclerosis?
  - Does the patient have any clues to gastrointestinal disease that are immediately apparent, eg a stoma?
  - What is the patient's colour, eg pale, cyanosed, jaundiced, ruddy complexion?
- Ask the patient to cough and then to lift their head off the bed. Note any herniae or divarication of rectus abdominis.

Hands

- Take the patient's hands in yours and look for:
    - finger clubbing
    - anaemia of palmar creases
    - evidence of smoking
    - leuconychia (white nails)
    - palmar erythema
    - Dupuytren's contracture.
- Test for a liver flap (asterixis):
    - Ask the patient to put their arms straight out in front of them and fan their fingers apart. Passively extend the wrists with the arms outstretched. Involuntary flexion may be present in liver failure.

Face

- Scan the eyes and face and look for:
    - xanthelasma
    - corneal arcus.
- Inspect the conjunctivae for anaemia, and look at the sclera for jaundice.
- Look in the mouth for ulcers. Note the hydration of the tongue. Subtly smell the breath for hepatic fetor (smells like stale urine/ammonia), diabetic ketoacidosis (sweet/acetone smell) or halitosis.
- Look for spider naevi on the face, arms and thorax.

Abdomen

- Look for:
    - swelling
    - distended veins
    - skin changes (eg bruising)
    - scars
    - herniae
    - pulsation
    - divarication of rectus muscles
    - stomas.
- Kneel down and look along the surface of the abdomen for peristaltic waves.

Make a point of looking in the flanks, eg for nephrectomy scars.

Palpation

Features to palpate
- General
- Liver
- Spleen
- Kidneys
- Bladder (when appropriate)
- Abdominal aorta

Before laying a finger on the patient's abdomen ask if there is any pain and, if so, leave the painful area until last. If you know there is painful area, you may consider it useful to employ diversion/distraction tactics. Talk to the patient about something you know they enjoy or will be chatty about (eg hobbies, grandchildren, pets) and they may forget about any pain you are inflicting.

General

This consists of superficial and deep palpation. For both, examine all nine regions of the abdomen in a systematic fashion (see diagram below). Palpate while kneeling at the side of the bed so that you are at the same level as the abdomen.

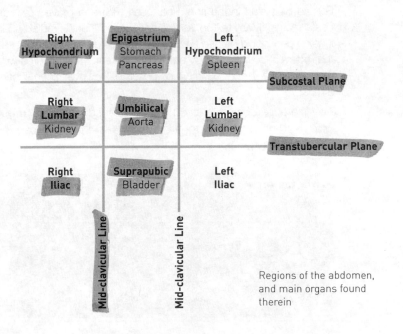

Regions of the abdomen, and main organs found therein

Ⓥ **Watch the patient's face for any sign of pain while you are palpating.**

Superficial palpation: With one hand flat on the abdomen, gently move the extended fingers up and down (by flexing at the MCP joints). You are trying to elicit:

- tenderness
- rigidity
- guarding

Deep palpation: This is usually performed with two hands (one on top of the other) and is used to detect masses and deep-seated pain. Some doctors prefer you to use one hand only, and simply to press harder than for superficial palpation.

Liver

For both the liver and spleen it is necessary to have respiration co-ordinated correctly with your palpation, since these organs move downwards, below the costal margin, during inspiration. To take advantage of this movement, use the expiratory phase to move your fingers into position and then hold them still during inspiration to try and feel the edge of these organs hit your fingers.

For the liver, start in the right iliac fossa (RIF) and move upwards to the costal margin. Many textbooks will recommend that the radial aspect of the index finger should be used, but it may be more effective to use the tips of the fingers of both hands. By doing this, a greater surface area will contact the liver, and a deeper push will be possible. However, short fingernails are a must!

After the edge of the liver has been established, percuss the upper and lower borders of the liver to confirm your findings. The upper border is normally in the right 5th intercostal space.

Liver features to be noted
- Size
- Surface (micro- or macronodular, ie tiny or large nodules)
- Edge (eg smooth, knobbly)
- Tenderness
- Consistency (eg hard, soft)
- Pulsatility

Enlargement of the liver/spleen should be recorded in centimetres (not finger-breadths).

Spleen

Again, start in the RIF, but this time work up to the left hypochondrium (since the spleen enlarges diagonally). The lateral tilt may then be performed. Ask the patient to turn slightly onto their right side, and examine the spleen again. Percuss the borders of the spleen if you suspect it is enlarged.

You should splint the left lower rib from behind, with your non-examining hand, to fix this mobile organ and make it more easily palpable anteriorly.

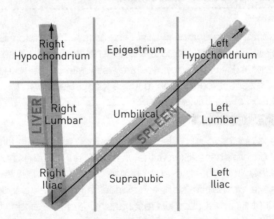

'Paths' taken in palpation of the liver and spleen

Kidneys

The kidneys are palpated with both hands (bimanual palpation). Some call this 'ballottment'. One hand should be placed on the abdomen, and should remain fixed; the other hand is placed posteriorly, and is used to 'flick' or 'bounce' the kidney between your hands.

Bladder (if indicated)

To palpate the bladder use the ulnar aspect of the hand and gently press over the suprapubic space – this is usually where an enlarged bladder will lie. This can be confirmed with light percussion. The dullness will extend to the pubic rim.

Abdominal aorta

You should place your fingers just above the umbilicus and push down firmly (but not too hard). The index and middle finger should be held together as one unit. An abdominal aortic aneurysm will usually make your fingers move upwards (pulsatile movement) and outwards (expansile movement).

The abdominal aorta may be palpated in some normal individuals and will feel pulsatile only.

Percuss the abdomen

Percussion should be carried out only when necessary – for example, with a suspected swollen abdomen.

Percuss the abdomen in all nine areas (see Respiratory System chapter for details on how to percuss). Note whether the percussion note is dull or resonant. By percussing, you are also testing for rebound tenderness. This is present if percussion causes pain. Rebound tenderness indicates irritation of the peritoneum.

Test for shifting dullness

Place one of your hands on the abdomen with the fingers pointed towards the patient's head. Start at the umbilicus, and percuss across the abdomen laterally until you find any change in the sound. It is likely to go from resonant to dull. This change signifies a border between air (resonant) and fluid (dull). The reason it is resonant in the centre of the abdomen is that air is present within loops of bowel, causing them to float on any fluid. Fluid goes to the flanks as gravity dictates.

Mark the border at which you found the change in sound, before asking the patient to roll towards you onto their right-hand side.

Percuss again and re-establish the area where the change from resonant to dull occurs. If fluid is present, the border will have changed as the fluid moves. The dullness has shifted, and the test is positive.

Test for a fluid thrill

Ask the patient to put the ulnar edge of one of their hands in the centre of the abdomen, orientated in a head-to-toe direction (this is done to prevent the movement of fat that may feel like a thrill).

Now flick the abdomen on one side, while keeping your other hand on the other side of the abdomen. If you feel a thrill, it is due to movement through the fluid.

To understand this concept, fill a balloon half-full with water and tap one side whilst feeling the other side. You can feel the ripple of the water and, unlike in the abdomen, you can see it too!

Auscultate the abdomen

This is done largely to hear bowel sounds, of which there are four types:

> **Types of bowel sounds**
> - Normal
> - Absent (with ileus)
> - Borborygmi (with increased peristalsis)
> - Tinkling (with obstruction)

Listen in the following areas (see diagram):
- Above the umbilicus – for bruits in the abdominal aorta
- 2 cm lateral to the umbilicus on both sides – for bruits in the renal arteries
- Over the liver – for a rub
- Over the spleen – for a rub.

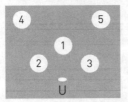

Positions for auscultation for bruits:
U = umbilicus; 1 = abdominal aorta;
2 & 3 = renovascular; 4 = liver; 5 = spleen

Thank the patient

Turn and face the examiner

State that you would like to complete the examination by:
- examining the groins and hernial orifices
- examining the external genitalia (see pages 127, 130)
- performing a rectal examination (see page 133)
- palpating the supraclavicular nodes, especially on the left-hand side, if you suspect that the patient may have an abdominal tumour. This is because tumours may spread along the lymphatic duct to this location
- observing the temperature chart
- performing urinalysis.

Examiners' favourites

Q Name some causes of a distended abdomen.

A The six Fs: fat, faeces, fluid, flatus, fetus (in females), flipping great tumour.

Q How would you differentiate between a splenic and a renal mass clinically?

A The spleen has notched edge; you cannot get 'above' the spleen; the spleen descends towards right iliac fossa on inspiration; the spleen is not ballottable; the spleen is dull to percussion.

Summary

ICE
▼
Inspect from the end of the bed
▼
Inspect the hands
▼
Inspect the face
▼
Inspect the abdomen
▼
Superficial palpation of the abdomen
▼
Deep palpation of the abdomen
▼
Palpate for a liver
▼
Palpate for a spleen
▼
Palpate for kidneys
▼
Palpate for a bladder (if indicated)
▼
Palpate for the abdominal aorta
▼
Percuss the abdomen if appropriate
▼
Auscultate the abdomen
▼
Thank the patient
▼
Turn and face the examiner

ICE

- Introduce yourself.
- Consent the patient for the examination.
- Expose the necessary parts of the body and position the patient. The face and neck should be exposed, and the patient should be sitting opposite you on a chair if possible.

Examination

Inspection

From the end of the bed

- Look around the bed for clues, eg details of a special diet on the wall if the patient has swallowing problems.
- Scan the patient from head to toe, and note:
  - Does the patient look well or unwell?
  - Does the patient have any obvious conditions, eg Parkinson's disease?

> A good way of remembering the examination is to work your way through each nerve in turn, and assess sensory function, and motor function where appropriate.

Cranial nerve	Sensory function/motor function/both
I	Sensory
II	Sensory
III	Motor
IV	Motor
V	Both
VI	Motor
VII	Motor
VIII	Sensory
IX	Both
X	Both
XI	Motor
XII	Motor

Cranial nerve I (olfactory nerve)

- Usually, simply asking if the patient has noticed a problem with smelling or tasting foods is sufficient.
- Formal testing requires using an aromatic material (such as orange peel or coffee granules) to test the patient's perception and identification.

V **Test both nostrils separately.**

Cranial nerve II (optic nerve) (see eye examination for further details)

- Inspect the eye and note pupil size, shape and equality between sides.
- Assess direct and consensual pupil reactions to light and accommodation.
- Test visual acuity.
- Test colour vision.
- Test visual fields by confrontation.
- Examine the fundus with a direct ophthalmoscope.

Cranial nerves III, IV and VI (oculomotor, trochlear and abducens nerves)

V **These three nerves are tested together due to their similar functions.**

- Inspect the eyelid position for ptosis (drooping). Look at the position of the upper lid relative to the iris on both sides.
- Test eye movements (see eye examination).
- If testing the third nerve in isolation, test the pupillary responses as described earlier (since this nerve is involved in these responses also).
- Test for strabismus (squint) by performing the cover test (see eye examination).
- Test for nystagmus. Ask the patient to fix on your fingertip. Hold their head steady so that movement of the eye occurs. Move your finger 30° in each of the eight directions shown in the diagram, and hold it steady in this position. Watch closely for deviation of the eyes. If nystagmus is present, note the direction of the fast phase and the position of gaze in which it is maximal. (NB. If the eyes deviate slowly to the right and then quickly to the left, the direction of nystagmus is 'to the left'.)

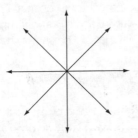

Directions in which to test
for nystagmus

Cranial nerve V (trigeminal nerve)

- Test the corneal reflex. Ask the patient to look directly in front. Using a wisp of cotton wool, approach the eye from the side and touch the cornea gently. The eyelids should blink. Test this on both sides.

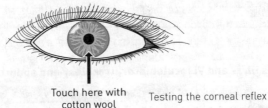

Touch here with
cotton wool

Testing the corneal reflex

- Test facial sensation. Ask the patient to close their eyes and to acknowledge when they sense you touching the face. Test soft touch (with cotton wool) and pinprick sensation. Test the three divisions of the nerve on both sides by testing sensation above the eyebrows, below the eyes and on the mandible, as shown in the diagram.

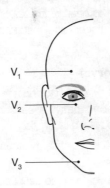

V_1

V_2

V_3

The three divisions of the
trigeminal nerve

- Test for a jaw jerk reflex. Ask the patient to open the mouth. Rest your index finger just below the lower lip, and strike your finger gently with the patellar hammer. A positive jaw jerk is present if the mandible 'jerks' upwards.
- Ask the patient to clench and unclench their teeth while palpating the masseter and temporalis muscles.
- Test the power of jaw opening and closing by asking the patient to resist while you attempt to close the opened jaw, and open the closed jaw.
- Test the power of jaw deviation. Ask the patient to open the mouth, deviate the jaw to one side and try to hold it in that position. The examiner should try to push the jaw back into the central position. Repeat with the jaw deviated towards the other side.

Cranial nerve VII (facial nerve)

- It is usually acceptable to assess taste by asking the patient whether a change in the taste of food has been noticed. If taste in the anterior two-thirds of the tongue is to be formally assessed, ask the patient to stick out the tongue and to distinguish between salt and sugar. Test both sides of the tongue independently, and ask the patient to identify the taste before the tongue is retracted into the mouth.
- Test facial movements by asking the patient to frown and to show their teeth.

> Testing the ability to frown is a good way to distinguish between upper and lower motor neurone lesions of this nerve. In a lower motor neurone problem, this ability is lost on the side of the affected nerve.

- Test the power of facial movement by asking the patient to close the eyes tightly and to resist your trying to open them. You should also attempt to part the patient's lips with your fingers after instructing them to try to keep the mouth closed.

Cranial nerve VIII (vestibulocochlear nerve)

- Crudely examine the patient's hearing using the whisper test. If the whisper test picks up an abnormality, assess hearing further using Rinné's and Weber's tests (see ear examination).
- If this nerve is being assessed in isolation, nystagmus should be tested for as described earlier.
- Balance should be tested if indicated (see peripheral nervous system).

Cranial nerves IX and X (glossopharyngeal and vagus nerves)

These nerves are assessed together.

- Note the patient's voice and ability to cough.
- Ask the patient to swallow some water and note any nasal regurgitation.
- Shine a light in the mouth and ask the patient to say 'Ah'. Note the position of the uvula (ie central or deviated to one side).
- Test for a gag reflex by gently touching both sides of the oropharynx with a tongue depressor and compare sensitivity and degree of palatal contraction between sides.

Cranial nerve XI (accessory nerve)

- Inspect the sternomastoid muscles and feel their bulk.
- Ask the patient to look over each shoulder in turn and try to hold the head in that position while you attempt to turn the head back towards the mid-line.
- Test both muscles together by asking the patient to bring the chin to the chest and to resist your movement as you try to push the head up again.
- Test the trapezius muscles by asking the patient to hold the shoulders in a shrugged position, while you attempt to push them down.

Cranial nerve XII (hypoglossal nerve)

- Ask the patient to stick out their tongue. Inspect the tongue and assess movement and any deviation.
- Test power by asking the patient to press out on the cheek with the tongue while you attempt to press it back towards the midline.

Thank the patient

Turn and face the examiner

Examiners' favourites

Q How would you distinguish clinically between an upper motor
neurone and lower motor neurone seventh cranial nerve palsy?

A Ask the patient to wrinkle their forehead. This movement will be lost
on the affected side when a lower motor neurone lesion is present.
With an upper motor neurone lesion, this movement will be
preserved, although the other muscles of facial expression will
generally be weak.

Q List four causes of a third cranial nerve palsy.

A Trauma, posterior communicating artery aneurysm, nasopharyngeal
tumour, diabetes mellitus.

Summary

ICE

▼

Inspect from the end of the bed

▼

Examine the cranial nerves in turn

▼

Thank the patient

▼

Turn and face the examiner

This system has lots to be examined. Learn the headings first, and then fill in the details.

If the patient reports a problem on one side, the normal side should be assessed first.

Components of PNS examination

- ICE
- Inspection
- Tone
- Power
- Co-ordination
- Reflexes
- Sensation

ICE

- Introduce yourself.
- Consent the patient for the examination.
- Expose the necessary parts of the body and position the patient. Sleeves should be rolled up to expose the arms. The legs and thighs should also be exposed. Blankets should be used to preserve patients' dignity. Position the back of the bed at 45° to the horizontal.

Examination

It is critical that you compare sides as you go along.

Inspection

From the end of the bed

- Look around the bed for clues, eg walking stick, wheelchair.
- Scan the patient from head to toe, and note:
  - Does the patient look well or unwell?
  - Does the patient have any obvious conditions, eg are they not moving one side of the body?
  - Does the patient have any clues to neurological disease that are immediately apparent, eg an involuntary movement, or a typical facial appearance?

Upper and lower limbs

Look for the following:

- Tremor
- Muscle wasting
- Muscle hypertrophy
- Asymmetry
- Abnormal posture
- Fasciculation (abnormal involuntary contraction of muscle fibres). If fasciculation is not obvious, you may gently flick the main muscle groups with your index finger and watch closely. It may take over 1 minute to demonstrate fasciculation, but this time should be cut short in an examination setting.

Perform the pronator drift test

Ask the patient to hold their arms out at around 135° to the body, with the palms facing up and the fingers spread apart. The patient should then close their eyes. If one arm drops and pronates (palms turn to face the floor), the test is positive, indicating that a pyramidal weakness is present.

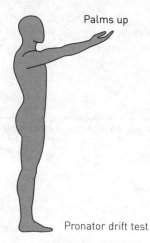

Palms up

Pronator drift test

Assess tone

Ask the patient if they have any pain in the limb you are going to test, and bear that in mind.

Upper limb

Passively move the limb through all shoulder movements, then progress to elbow flexion and extension. Next, hold the patient's hand as if you were going to shake hands, and test pronation and supination. You should also quickly perform wrist extension and flexion as well as finger movements. Try to assess whether the tone is normal, increased or decreased.

Classification of increased tone
- Lead pipe (increased tone throughout the movement)
- Cog wheel (ratchet-like movement)
- Clasp knife (increased tone which suddenly gives way)

Lower limb

Ask the patient to lie on a couch. Firstly, with the leg straight, roll the leg from side to side. Next, lift up the leg just above the knee, and allow it to drop back onto the bed. Normally, the leg should drop easily back into position. With increased tone, the lower leg may move abnormally. Check the tone at the ankle joint by extending and flexing. Finally, flex and extend the toes.

Test for clonus

This sign is indicative of increased tone. Flex and extend the foot a few times gently, and then suddenly dorsiflex (point towards the head) the foot at the ankle joint. Hold the foot in this position for several seconds. If clonus is present, you will feel the foot pushing back against your hand in a regular fashion for more than five 'beats'. A few beats of clonus can be normal.

Test power

It is possible to test power in every muscle group, but this is not done routinely. The major muscle groups described below are always tested to assess their power. When deciding how powerful a muscle group is, the Medical Research Council grading system is used.

Medical Research Council power grading system
Grade 0: No muscular contraction
Grade 1: Muscle contraction but no movement
Grade 2: Movement with gravity eliminated
Grade 3: Movement against gravity
Grade 4: Movement against gravity and resistance
Grade 5: Normal power

A particular difficulty when testing power is getting the patient to do what you want them to do. This is best overcome by practising the technique and working out what you will say to the patient beforehand. All testing of muscle power essentially consists of getting the patient to try to resist your force.

When performing these tests you should compare sides as you go along: test right shoulder abduction then left shoulder abduction, and so on. If the muscle group is weak, you may have to test the movement with gravity eliminated. This may require the patient to change body position, eg they should lie on their side for hip flexion and extension.

Upper limb

Shoulder abduction

Ask the patient to abduct the shoulders to 90° and to hold the arms in that position while you attempt to push the arms down against the body.

Testing power of shoulder abduction

Patient's effort   Patient's effort

Examiner's effort   Examiner's effort

Elbow flexion

Ask the patient to flex the elbows and to keep them flexed while you attempt to straighten the arm.

Testing power of elbow flexion

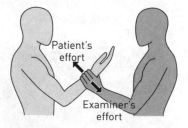

Patient's effort

Examiner's effort

Elbow extension

Ask the patient to keep their arm straight while you try to bend it.

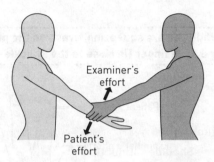

Testing power of elbow extension

Examiner's effort

Patient's effort

Wrist flexion

Ask the patient to keep their wrist flexed while you try to extend it.

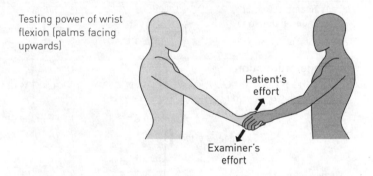

Testing power of wrist flexion (palms facing upwards)

Patient's effort

Examiner's effort

Wrist extension

Ask the patient to keep their wrist extended while you try to flex it.

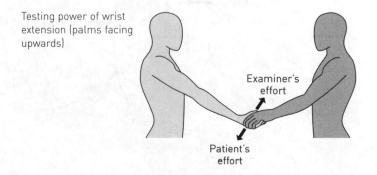

Testing power of wrist extension (palms facing upwards)

Examiner's effort

Patient's effort

Finger abduction

Ask the patient to fan out their fingers while you try to squeeze them back together.

While you are squeezing, press on the proximal phalanx of the index and little finger (ie close to the knuckle).

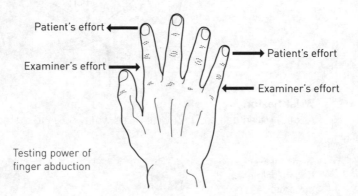

Patient's effort ←
Examiner's effort →
Patient's effort →
Examiner's effort ←

Testing power of finger abduction

Finger adduction

Ask the patient to hold a piece of paper between their index and middle fingers while you try to remove it.

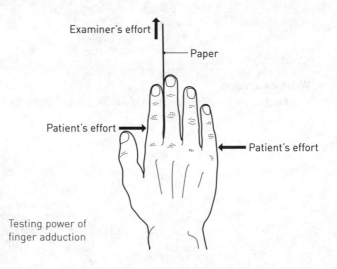

Examiner's effort
Paper
Patient's effort →
Patient's effort ←

Testing power of finger adduction

Lower limb

Hip flexion

Ask the patient to keep their legs straight and to raise them off the bed. You should then press down on the leg above knee level and attempt to press the leg back onto the bed.

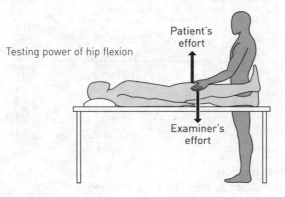

Testing power of hip flexion

Patient's effort

Examiner's effort

Hip extension

Slip your hand under the patient's leg, just above the knee. Ask the patient to press your hand into the bed, while you try to lift the patient's leg off the bed.

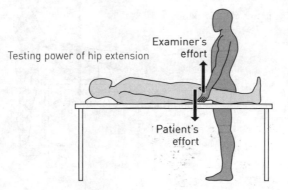

Testing power of hip extension

Examiner's effort

Patient's effort

Knee flexion

Ask the patient to keep their knee flexed while you try to extend it.

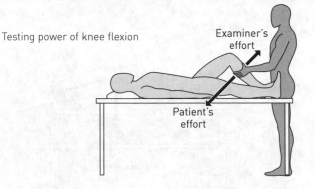

Testing power of knee flexion

Knee extension

Ask the patient to keep their knee extended while you try to flex it. It is necessary to support the patient's leg when testing knee extension.

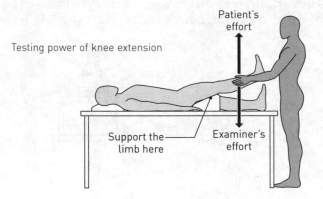

Testing power of knee extension

Ankle dorsiflexion

Ask the patient to keep their foot pointed towards their head while you try to plantar flex it.

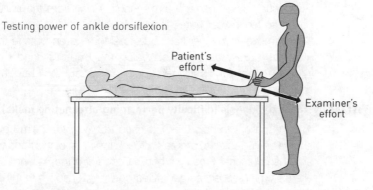

Testing power of ankle dorsiflexion

Patient's effort

Examiner's effort

Plantar flexion

Ask the patient to keep their foot pointed away from their head while you try to dorsiflex it.

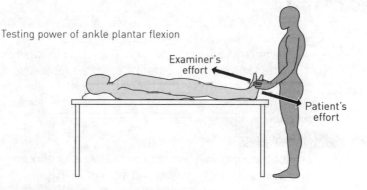

Testing power of ankle plantar flexion

Examiner's effort

Patient's effort

It is a good idea to feel the muscle group that you are testing while you are assessing it. For example, if you are testing elbow flexion, rest one hand on the bulk of the biceps muscle while the other hand attempts to straighten the arm. This will catch out the patient who is not making an attempt to move!

Test co-ordination

These all test cerebellar function.

Finger–nose test

Hold your index finger one arm's length away from the patient. Ask the patient to touch your finger, then their nose, then your finger, and so on. Slowly, move your finger from side to side, and encourage the patient to move as quickly as possible. Watch the patient's hand closely for an intention tremor, dysmetria (pointing past the target) or ataxia (inco-ordination). Repeat this with the other hand.

Test for dysdiadochokinesis (difficulty performing alternating tasks)

Ask the patient to hold their left hand out with the palm upwards. They should be instructed to alternately touch the palm of this hand with the palm and then dorsum of the right hand. Encourage the patient to perform this alternating movement as quickly as possible, ensuring that the two hands are completely separated between movements. A difficulty in performing this action may indicate dysdiadochokinesis. This test should then be conducted on the other side.

Heel–shin test

Examination of co-ordination in the lower limb involves asking the patient to lie out flat on the couch. The heel of one foot should be placed on the contralateral shin, just below the knee. The patient should then run the heel down this leg towards the ankle. When this movement is complete, the patient should lift the heel off the leg and replace it on the upper shin again. This series of movements should be repeated several times, before being done on the other side.

Gait and Romberg's test

Ask the patient to walk and note any instability or abnormal movements. Also assess the length of stride and the width of base.

Have the patient stand with their heels together with their eyes open, then closed. Instability on closing the eyes (Romberg test-positive) is indicative of a problem with proprioception.

Test reflexes

When testing reflexes, it is important that the patient is relaxed. Encourage them to let the limb 'go loose' or 'floppy' when you are testing. Use the full pendulum action of the tendon hammer by holding it near the end. Allow the hammer to fall under its own weight to ensure consistency between tests. Before striking, line up the hammer on the skin over the tendon.

Upper limb

Biceps reflex

Ask the patient to flex their elbow to 90°, and to rest their forearm on their abdomen. Feel for the biceps tendon with one hand and rest your thumb on top of it. Strike your thumb with the patellar hammer, and watch the biceps muscle for any contraction. Go on to test the other side.

Triceps reflex

Have the patient position their arm as before, and strike the triceps tendon directly, just above the olecranon process. Watch for contraction of the triceps muscle. Repeat on the other side.

Supinator reflex

Keep the patient's arm in the same position. Rest your thumb or finger over the lower radius on the extensor aspect of the arm, and strike with the tendon hammer. Watch for movement in the arm.

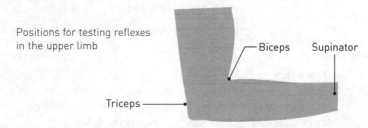

Positions for testing reflexes in the upper limb

Biceps Supinator

Triceps

Finger jerk reflex

Take all four of the patient's fingers loosely in your hand. Strike **your** fingers once with the patellar hammer as shown in the diagram. If this reflex is present, you will feel the patient's fingers flexing against yours.

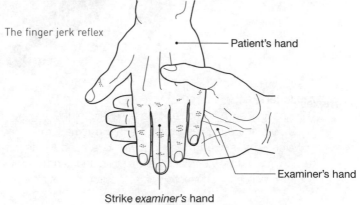

The finger jerk reflex

Patient's hand

Examiner's hand

Strike *examiner's* hand
in this position

Hoffman reflex

Support the middle phalanx of the patient's middle finger between your index and middle fingers. Flick the distal phalanx of this finger with your thumb. Watch for flexion of the patient's thumb. This may indicate increased reflexes, but is also present in some normal individuals.

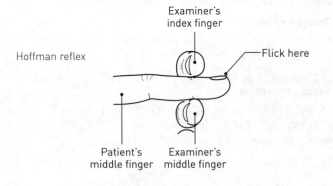

Examiner's
index finger

Hoffman reflex

Flick here

Patient's   Examiner's
middle finger   middle finger

Lower limb

Knee jerk

Support the patient's legs by placing your arm under their bent knees (bent to about 135°). Strike the patellar tendon just below the knee on the patellar tendon. Watch for contraction of the quadriceps muscles.

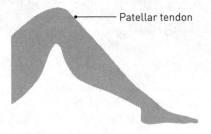

Position for testing the
knee jerk reflex

Patellar tendon

Ankle jerk

With the knees still flexed, ask the patient to let their legs fall down to the sides so that the leg lies on the bed (ie externally rotate the hip). Press upwards on the sole of their foot with one hand to stretch the Achilles tendon and, with the other hand, strike the tendon with the patellar hammer. Watch for contraction of the gastrocnemius muscle.

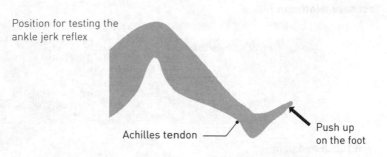

Position for testing the
ankle jerk reflex

Achilles tendon ——

Push up
on the foot

Plantar reflexes

Warn the patient that the test will be uncomfortable. Use a pointed object (eg a key – make sure it's not too sharp!) and, starting at the heel, run the point up the lateral border of the foot. Just below the toes run the point medially. This should be done very quickly. When you are doing the test, watch the patient's great toe carefully. Record the very first movement of this toe as either upwards or downwards.

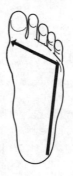

Direction used to test plantar
reflexes

If you are unable to elicit a tendon reflex, you should try again using a technique called 'reinforcement'. In either the upper or lower limb, ask the patient to clench their teeth hard just before you test for the reflex. In the lower limb, it is also possible to ask the patient to interlock the fingers of both hands together and then pull tight just before you test the reflex. If you are still unable to elicit the reflex after a couple of attempts with reinforcement, move on to the next stage in the examination, and record that you were unable to elicit the reflex.

Test sensation

Modalities of sensation

- Light touch
- Pain
- Two-point discrimination
- Temperature
- Vibration
- Joint position sense (proprioception)

Light touch and pain

Test light touch and pain together. Use a cotton-wool ball for light touch and a sharp point for pain. Show the patient the materials before you use them and touch the patient on the sternum with them so they can appreciate what they feel like.

Ask the patient to close their eyes, while you touch them with either the cotton wool or the point. The patient should identify which material is being used. Test each dermatome with both sensations in the limb being tested. Vary which material you touch the patient with to reduce the chance of them guessing correctly. If the patient is unable to distinguish between the two materials, touch them with both and ask if they can appreciate which one is sharper. If an abnormality is found, the distribution should be mapped out. You should record the position where the sensation returns to normal.

Two-point discrimination

Use two blunt points. Try to determine how closely you can touch the two points together on the patient's skin while the sensation is still recognised as being separate. If the points are too close, the patient will only be aware of being touched by a single point. The distance will vary depending on where the test is carried out, eg two points will be discriminated much closer on the fingertips than on the back.

Temperature

To test temperature, special bottles can be used. One should be filled with cold water and the other with warm water. The patient should be asked to identify which is hot and which is cold. In practice, these bottles are seldom available for use. You should therefore take a cold object (such as a metal tuning fork) and ask the patient if they can sense that it is cold.

Vibration sensation

A 128-Hz tuning fork is used to test vibration sensation. The fork should be struck and the non-vibrating end pressed against a bony prominence such as the medial malleolus. Ask the patient if they can feel the vibration. Then repeat the test several times, sometimes not striking the fork, and ask the patient to identify whether or not it is vibrating. If the patient is not able to identify the vibration, move more proximally on the limb.

Joint position sense

Joint position sense is first assessed in the thumb and great toe. Grasp the patient's digit just proximal to the distal interphalangeal joint at the sides (not above and below). Move the distal phalanx up and down, again holding onto the sides of the patient's finger, and explain to the patient what you are doing. Now, ask the patient to close their eyes, and identify whether you are moving the digit up or down. Repeat this several times to ensure that the patient is not guessing. If this sensation is intact, the examination can stop here. If it is impaired, move proximally and repeat the test in the next large joint, eg wrist/ankle.

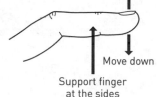

Technique used to assess proprioception

Move up

Move down

Support finger at the sides

Always remember to compare sides.

Thank the patient

Turn and face the examiner

> **Examiners' favourites**
>
> **Q** Which spinal roots are tested in the main reflex tests?
>
> **A** Biceps, C5, C6. Triceps, C6, C7, C8. Supinator, C6, C7. Knee, L2, L3, L4. Ankle, S1, S2
>
> **Q** In which parts of the spinal cord are the various modalities of sensation carried?
>
> **A** Pain, Spinothalamic tract. Temperature, Spinothalamic tract. Light touch Posterior column. Joint position sense, Posterior column (proprioception). Vibration, Posterior column. Two-point discrimination, Posterior column.

Summary

ICE
▼
Inspect from the end of the bed
▼
Inspect the upper and lower limbs
▼
Perform the pronator drift test
▼
Assess tone
▼
Test power
▼
Test co-ordination
▼
Test reflexes
▼
Test sensation
▼
Thank the patient
▼
Turn and face the examiner

The GALS screen is a musculoskeletal screening test that covers the essential aspects of many of the individual joint examinations.

ICE

- Introduce yourself.
- Consent the patient for the examination.
- Expose the necessary parts of the body and position the patient. Remove the shirt/blouse to expose the arms, shoulders and back. Brassieres should not be removed. Cover ladies with a blanket when not examining the chest. Trousers should also be removed to allow adequate inspection of the legs. The bed should be flat if the patient can tolerate it.

You should look for, and record, any abnormalities in any aspect of the screening test.

Examination

Inspection

From the end of the bed

- Look around the bed for clues to disease, eg walking stick, Zimmer frame.
- Scan the patient from head to toe, and note:
  - Does the patient look well or unwell?
  - Does the patient have any obvious conditions?
  - What is their body habitus, eg normal weight, cushingoid?
  - What is the patient's colour, eg pale, cyanosed, plethoric, ruddy complexion?

Three questions

- Have you any pain or stiffness in your muscles, joints or back?
- Can you dress yourself completely without any difficulty?
- Can you walk up and down stairs without any difficulty?

Gait

Ask the patient to walk to the other side of the room, turn, and walk back to you.

Spine

- Inspect the patient standing: from in front, the side and behind.
- Ask the patient to bend over and touch their toes, keeping the knees straight (lumbar flexion).

Estimate the amount of lumbar flexion by putting your fingers on adjacent vertebrae and noting the distance that they separate during flexion.

- Ask the patient to put 'their ear to their shoulder' on each side in turn (lateral cervical flexion).
- Squeeze the supraspinatus muscles – the positions are shown in the diagram.

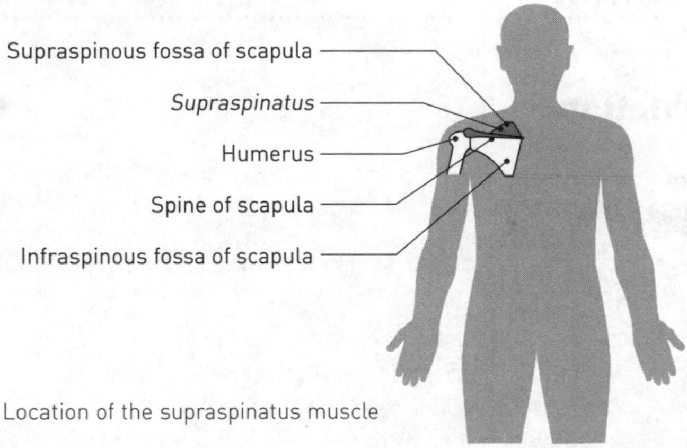

Supraspinous fossa of scapula
Supraspinatus
Humerus
Spine of scapula
Infraspinous fossa of scapula

Location of the supraspinatus muscle

Arms

- Inspect the patient's arms, with the elbows extended by the side in the anatomical position, as shown in the diagram opposite.

The position of the arms for inspection

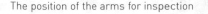

- Keeping the elbows by the side (so fixing them), ask the patient to flex the elbows to 90° and ask the patient to turn their palms towards the ceiling (supination), then down to the floor (pronation).
- Squeeze across the 1st–5th metacarpophalangeal (MCP) joints, and note any pain.
- Ask the patient to touch each finger, in turn, onto the thumb.
- Ask the patient to make a fist.
- Ask the patient to put their hands behind their head and to push the elbows backwards.

Legs

With the patient standing

- Inspect when standing – from the front, side and from behind (pay special attention to the popliteal fossa).

With the patient on the bed (see hip and knee examinations for further details)

- Inspect the legs close up.
- Feel the temperature of the knee by placing the back of your hand over the anterior aspect.
- Carry out the bulge test (with or without the patellar tap) for a fluid effusion in the knee.
- Ask the patient to put each heel up to their bottom (active knee and hip flexion).
- Passively flex the hip.
- While the hip is still flexed, test internal rotation passively.
- Extend the knee, keeping one hand over the patella to feel for crepitus.

- Squeeze across the 2nd–5th metatarsophalangeal (MTP) joints.
- Inspect the foot closely for callosities and other abnormalities. Look between the toes, at the metatarsal heads and at the heel.

Thank the patient

Turn and face the examiner

Summary

ICE

▼

Inspect from the end of the bed

▼

Ask three questions

▼

Assess gait

▼

Asses the spine

▼

Assess the arms

▼

Assess the legs

▼

Thank the patient

▼

Turn and face the examiner

SECTION 2
REGIONAL EXAMINATIONS

When a patient presents to a doctor, it is not always obvious which body system (or systems) is responsible for their symptoms. A systematic general inspection will guide your history-taking and further examination. All the examinations detailed in this book have a section where a general inspection of the patient should be performed from the end of the bed. The following points should be considered. Many of these features will be noted subconsciously when assessing a patient.

State of illness

- Where does the patient fit on a spectrum that ranges from well to close to death?

Colour

What colour is the patient? they may be:

- anaemic (pale)
- cyanotic: blue lips (central cyanosis) and/or extremities (peripheral cyanosis)
- jaundiced (yellow)
- uraemic (grey)
- flushed (pink)
- polycythaemic (ruddy)
- drug-induced pigmentation (eg, purple from chlorpromazine).

Odour

Does a smell greet you as you speak to the patient? Consider:

- recreational activities: alcohol, tobacco, marijuana
- hepatic fetor (stale urine/ammonia)
- uraemic fetor (mice)
- diabetic ketoacidosis (sweet/acetone)
- otherwise malodorous (excess sweating, poor hygiene).

Hydration and nutrition

- Gross dehydration, oedema?
- Cachectic, underweight, normal weight, overweight, obese?

Attire

- Well groomed or unkempt?
- Appropriately dressed for the time, place and environment?
- Spectacles/contact lenses/intraocular lenses?
- Hearing aid/cochlear implant?
- Laryngeal voice box?
- Walking aids: walking stick, Delta Rollator, Zimmer frame, white stick (if blind)?

Facial appearance

There are many specific facial signs; several are indicative of a particular disease process, for example:

- Malar flush (in mitral stenosis)
- Butterfly rash (in SLE)
- Temporalis wasting (in myotonic dystrophy)
- Lack of facial expression (Parkinson's disease)
- Moon face (Cushing's syndrome)
- Coarse features with a large mandible (acromegaly)
- Tight skin, pinched nose, small mouth (scleroderma).

Speech

There may be something unusual about how the patient talks, such as:

- Hoarseness (eg in laryngitis)
- 'Donald duck' speech (in pseudobulbar palsy)
- Dysarthria, dysphasia, dysphonia
- Educationally limited.

Position and posture

- Does the patient need to sit up or lie down?
- Is the patient in pain?
- Are there any involuntary or abnormal movements (tremor, tics, fasciculation, writhing)?
- Does the patient limp on entering the room?
- Is there abnormal kyphosis/lordosis/scoliosis?

Body structure

Inspect for the following:

- Mastectomy
- Amputation with or without prostheses
- False eye
- Toupée
- Tracheostomy
- Prominent dermatological conditions, eg port wine stain.

Objects and belongings

The following may be noticed beside the patient:

- 'Medic-Alert' bracelet
- Tobacco products
- Catheter bag on the edge of the bed
- Diabetic insulin pens, GTN spray, inhalers
- Sputum container. Note the colour of any sputum: white frothy (pulmonary oedema); green/yellow (infection); blood (haemoptysis)
- Nebuliser, oxygen mask/intranasal prongs, nutrient drinks
- Sleeping arrangements: 'ripple' bed, number of pillows, isolation room
- Evidence of hospital treatment, eg iv line in situ, chest drain, central venous line
- Signs around the bed, eg fluid restriction sign or swallowing precautions, MRSA status.

Hospital records

The following may be provided by nursing staff or by examiners in an assessment scenario.

- Temperature, pulse rate, blood pressure, oxygen saturations, respiratory rate, Glasgow Coma Scale, fluid input/output, weight, blood sugar, etc.

There are potentially many more features that you may notice on observing a patient during a medical consultation – this list is far from complete. Findings picked up in this way may help explain a good deal of the patient's symptomatology.

No clinical speciality has as many examinations or special tests as those in musculoskeletal medicine. In fact, sometimes there is more than one way of examining the same thing! Initially this may daze, bewilder and knock self-confidence but, once you establish a routine and practise your technique, all examinations can be done quickly and efficiently.

All these examinations follow the same overall format.

Examination format
- ICE
- Inspection
- Palpation
- Measure
- Move – active and passive
- Special tests
- Function

In an active test, the patient moves the limb.

In a passive test, the examiner moves the limb.

It is often helpful to demonstrate the movements that you would like the patient to make. This is much easier than having to describe each movement.

Measurements (if applicable) and special tests can come wherever you choose in the general routine of the examination, and should be done at the most convenient moment for both yourself and the patient. As long as you have a smooth, memorable system, it does not matter about the order.

Make sure you inspect any appropriate radiographs if available.

Ensure that you always examine both sides of the patient. If you are asked to examine a patient's right knee, for example, state that you would first like to examine the left knee for comparative purposes.

There is much more to the hand examination than merely examining the joints. This chapter details joint examination only. Refer to page 93 for the complete hand examination.

....

V **The examination of the hand begins as soon as you meet the patient – when you shake hands. A tremor, painful joints, warmth, weakness or lack of digits are just a few points you may note.**

....

ICE

- Introduce yourself.
- Consent the patient for the examination.
- Expose the necessary parts of the body and position the patient. Roll the patient's sleeves up to the elbow, and place the hands on a white pillow. The patient can be seated for this examination.

Examination

Inspection

From the end of the bed

- Look around the bed for clues, eg occupational therapy aids for holding cups and unscrewing lids.
- Scan the patient from head to toe, and note:
  - Does the patient look well or unwell?
  - Does the patient have any obvious conditions, eg systemic sclerosis, rheumatoid arthritis?
- What is the patient's appearance? Eg cushingoid due to steroids.

Hands

- Inspect the dorsal and palmar surfaces. Look for:
  - scars
  - hand posture
  - skin changes
  - deformities (note the pattern of any deformity)
  - subluxation
  - muscle wasting (especially at thenar/hypothenar eminences)
  - swelling – bony, soft or fluid (note the distribution of the swelling).

- Inspect the nails. Look for:
  - pitting
  - onycholysis
  - subungual hyperkeratosis
  - nail-fold infarcts.

Ⓥ Inspect the elbows for clues to the cause of joint pathology.

Palpation

Gently palpate around the wrist and all the small joints of the hand: carpal bones; carpometacarpal (CMC), metacarpophalangeal (MCP), proximal interphalangeal (PIP) and distal interphalangeal (DIP) joints, as well as the interphalangeal (IP) joint in the thumb.

Ⓥ Make a point of carefully palpating the anatomical snuffbox, since scaphoid pathology is easily missed.

At each joint, feel for:

- temperature
- swelling
- tenderness
- bony abnormalities.

Squeeze across the MCP joints and ask about tenderness.

Joints in the hand: proximal
interphalangeal joints (PIP);
distal interphalangeal joints (DIP);
metacarpophalangeal joints (MCP);
interphalangeal joint of the thumb (IP)

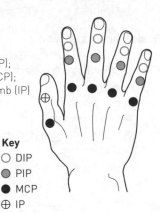

Key
○ DIP
◑ PIP
● MCP
⊕ IP

Active movements

Before testing hand movements, check the patient has good shoulder function as, without it, hand function is limited. To do this, ask the patient to place the hands behind the head, with elbows well back.

If it is apparent that a patient has limited movement in the hand joints, do not ask them to perform movements again and again. It can be distressing to have limited hand function as it reduces one's ability to carry out activities of daily living.

Wrist

Pronation and supination

The patient's elbows must be fixed and held pinned into the side.

- Ask the patient to turn their palms towards the floor (pronation), and then towards the sky (supination). Remember: supinate to the sky!

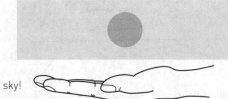

Supinate to the sky!

Flexion and extension

Ask the patient to form the prayer (extension) and inverse prayer (flexion) positions. For the inverse prayer position, put the dorsal (back of hand) surfaces of the hands together.

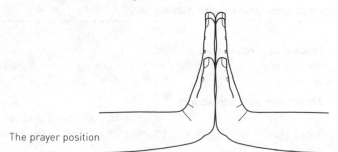

The prayer position

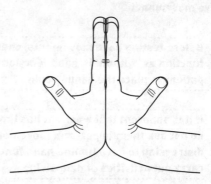

The inverse prayer position

Abduction and adduction

Fix the forearm just above the wrist (to ensure movement is occurring at the wrist, not the shoulder), before asking the patient to move the hands apart (abduction) and then together (adduction).

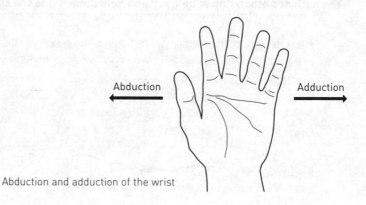

← Abduction   Adduction →

Abduction and adduction of the wrist

Thumb

Place the dorsal surface of the hand flat on the pillow, and fix the wrist to prevent interference with movement.

Flexion and extension

Ask the patient to curl in their thumb (flexion), and then straighten it out (extension).

Abduction and adduction

Ask the patient to keep the thumb straight, then to move the thumb away from the palm (abduction), and then back towards it (adduction).

Opposition

Ask the patient to touch the tip of each finger with the tip of the thumb of the same hand.

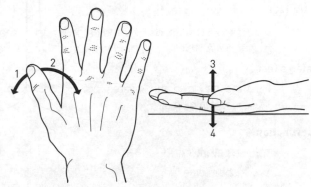

Some thumb movements: (1 = extension; 2 = flexion;
3 = abduction; 4 = adduction)

Fingers

Flexion and extension

Ask the patient to make a fist (flexion) and then to open it out (extension).

Abduction and adduction

Ask the patient to keep the hands in a horizontal plane. They should spread their fingers apart (abduction) and then back together (adduction).

Grips

Ask the patient to squeeze your finger tightly. You may also wish to test:

- precision grip (rolling a coin between finger and thumb)
- ball grip (picking up a tennis ball)
- flat pinch (holding a key between forefinger and thumb)
- writing (holding a pen)
- hook (carrying a suitcase)
- unscrewing (unscrewing the lid of a jar).

Passive movements

Work through all the above movements again. This time move the hand or digit yourself rather than asking the patient to perform the movement.

Be sure that you are not causing the patient any pain when testing passive movements.

Special tests

The following are two tests for carpal tunnel syndrome. Perform these only if the patient has symptoms suggestive of this diagnosis.

Tinel's test

Percuss for 30 seconds over the carpal tunnel on the flexor aspect of the wrist to try to elicit the symptoms of carpal tunnel syndrome.

Phalen's test

Hold the hands in the inverse prayer position for a minute to try to reproduce symptoms.

Test function

Ask the patient to:

• write their name

• fasten and undo a button

• pour and drink a glass of water.

Thank the patient

Turn and face the examiner

Examiners' favourites

Q What are the common features of osteoarthritis in the hands?

A Heberden's nodes (at the DIPs), Bouchard's nodes (at the PIPs), squaring of the hands.

Q What are the common features of rheumatoid arthritis in the hands?

A Radial deviation of the wrist, ulnar deviation of the fingers, Z-shaped thumb, boutonnière deformity, swan-neck deformity.

Summary

ICE

▼

Inspect from the end of the bed

▼

Inspect the hands

▼

Palpate the wrist and hand joints

▼

Test active movements at the wrist, thumb and fingers

▼

Test passive movements at the wrist, thumb and fingers

▼

Perform Tinel's test (if applicable)

▼

Perform Phalen's test (if applicable)

▼

Test function

▼

Thank the patient

▼

Turn and face the examiner

ICE

- Introduce yourself.
- Consent the patient for the examination.
- Expose the necessary part of the body and position the patient. The whole arm should be exposed – ask the patient to remove their top. Use a blanket to preserve female patients' dignity. The patient should be standing.

Examination

Inspection

From the end of the bed

- Look around the bed for clues, eg occupational therapy aids for holding cups and unscrewing lids.
- Scan the patient from head to toe, and note:
  - Does the patient look well or unwell?
  - Does the patient have any obvious conditions, eg psoriasis or tophaceours gout?

Elbows

- Inspect from in front, the side and behind. Look for:
  - scars
  - skin changes
  - deformities
  - muscle wasting
  - swelling – bony, soft, fluid, or skin nodules.

Palpation

- Gently palpate around the elbow joints. Feel for bony landmarks, and carefully palpate any skin nodules.
- At each joint, feel for:
  - temperature
  - swelling
  - tenderness
  - bony abnormalities.

Active movements

Before testing elbow movements, check the patient has good shoulder function as, without it, elbow function is limited. To do this, ask the patient to place the hands behind the head, with elbows well back.

Flexion and extension

> The patient's elbows must be fixed and held pinned into the side.

Ask the patient to bend their arms as much as possible (flexion), and then to straighten them out (extension). Note whether or not the patient is able to fully extend the elbows.

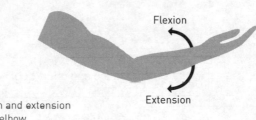

Flexion

Extension

Flexion and extension
of the elbow

Passive movements

Work through all the above movements again. This time, move the arm yourself rather than asking the patient to perform the movement.

> Be sure that you are not causing the patient any pain when testing passive movements.

Test function

Ask the patient to:

• pour and drink a glass of water

• put on a cardigan or coat.

Thank the patient

Turn and face the examiner

Examiners' favourites

Q Give a differential diagnosis for a lump on the extensor aspect of the elbow.

A Sebaceous cyst, a bursa, a gouty tophus, a rheumatoid nodule, a bony swelling.

Q List some causes of a skin rash on the extensor aspect of the elbow.

A Psoriasis, eczema, dermatitis herpetiformis.

Summary

ICE
▼
Inspect from the end of the bed
▼
Inspect the elbows
▼
Palpate the elbow joints
▼
Test active movements
▼
Test passive movements
▼
Test function
▼
Thank the patient
▼
Turn and face the examiner

The shoulder, unlike most other major joints, is made up of multiple joints that cannot be tested in isolation.

ICE

- **I**ntroduce yourself.
- **C**onsent the patient for the examination.
- **E**xpose the necessary parts of the body and position the patient. The whole arm should be exposed – ask the patient to remove any covering tops. Use a blanket to preserve female patients' dignity. The patient should be standing.

Watching the patient undress may demonstrate functional impairment resulting from shoulder pathology.

Examination

Inspection

From the end of the bed

- Look around the bed for clues, eg comb extensions, long shoe horns.
- Scan the patient from head to toe, and note:
  - Does the patient look well or unwell?
  - Does the patient have any obvious conditions, eg ankylosing spondylitis?

Shoulders

Inspect from in front, the side and behind. Look for:

- asymmetry
- muscle wasting (especially of the deltoid)
- abnormal posture
- swelling
- scars
- bruising
- deformity
- whether the shoulders are level or not.

Also inspect the axillae.

Palpation

Stand in front of the patient and palpate the following structures, in this order:

- Sternoclavicular joint
- Clavicle
- Acromioclavicular joint
- Acromial process
- Head of humerus
- Coracoid process
- Spine of scapula (from behind)
- Greater tuberosity of humerus.

Observe the patient's face for any tenderness and feel for swelling. Use the dorsum of your hand to feel the temperature over each shoulder.

Measure

Assess the deltoid bulk by measuring the circumference at the top of both arms.

Active movements

Flexion and extension

Ask the patient to flex the elbow to 90°, and move the arm upwards until the fist points backwards (flexion), then move the arm backwards as far as possible (extension).

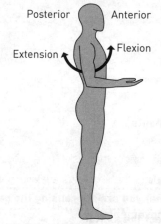

Posterior   Anterior

Extension   Flexion

Flexion and extension of the shoulder

Abduction and adduction

With the elbow fully extended, ask the patient to bring the arm away from the body until the fingertips point to the ceiling (abduction), and then to swing the arm across the trunk (adduction).

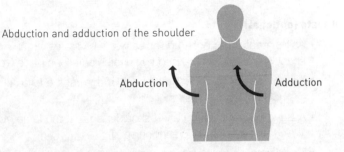

Abduction and adduction of the shoulder

Abduction   Adduction

External and internal rotation

With the elbows fixed to 90° and pinned into the side, have the patient move the forearms in an arc-like motion, thus separating the hands (external rotation), and bringing them together (internal rotation).

Ensure the elbows are kept tightly into the sides.

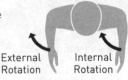

Internal and external rotation of the shoulder (viewed from above)

External   Internal
Rotation   Rotation

Passive movements

Work through all the above movements again. This time, move the arm yourself rather than asking the patient to perform the movement.

Be sure that you are not causing the patient any pain when testing passive movements.

....

When testing passive abduction and adduction, use one of your hands to fix the scapula so that you can account for any movement here. Movement of the scapula can give the false impression of movement at the shoulder.

....

Special tests (optional)

- Ask the patient to push against a wall with flat palms and observe the scapulae for winging (caused by serratus anterior muscle weakness).
- Ask the patient to abduct the shoulder against the force of your hands (painful in supraspinatus tendonitis).
- Ask the patient to shrug each shoulder against the force of your hands (difficult in pathology of cranial nerve XI).
- Test the sensation over the 'regimental badge area' on the skin over the deltoid muscle (to assess axillary nerve sensory function).
- You may wish to test the circulation to the upper limb – palpate the brachial and radial arteries.

Test function

Ask the patient to:

- put their hands behind their head with the elbows as far back as possible
- scratch the centre of the back as far up as possible
- put on a coat.

Thank the patient

Turn and face the examiner

Examiners' favourites

Q Where might shoulder pain be referred from?

A Shoulder joint, axilla, cervical spine, under the diaphragm, the heart.

Q Which joints make up the shoulder girdle?

A Glenohumeral, acromioclavicular, sternoclavicular, thoracoscapular.

Summary

ICE
▼
Inspect from the end of the bed
▼
Inspect the shoulders
▼
Palpate the shoulders
▼
Measure the upper arm circumference
▼
Test active movements at the shoulder
▼
Test passive movements at the shoulder
▼
Test for serratus anterior weakness (optional)
▼
Test for supraspinatus tendonitis (optional)
▼
Test the power of shoulder shrugging (optional)
▼
Test for regimental badge area sensory loss (optional)
▼
Palpate the brachial and radial arteries (optional)
▼
Test function
▼
Thank the patient
▼
Turn and face the examiner

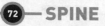

The spine can be divided into three regions for the purpose of clinical examination: cervical, thoracic and lumbar.

ICE

- **I**ntroduce yourself.
- **C**onsent the patient for the examination.
- **E**xpose the necessary parts of the body and position the patient. Remove the shirt or blouse. Brassieres should not be removed. The patient should be standing.

Examination

Inspection

From the end of the bed

- Look around the bed for clues, eg a wheelchair.
- Scan the patient from head to toe, and note:
  - Does the patient look well or unwell?
  - Does the patient have any obvious conditions, eg Dowager's hump?
  - Does the patient have an unusual posture?

Spine

- Inspection should take place from:
  - behind
  - in front
  - the side: sitting and standing.
- Look for:
  - abnormal kyphosis (convex curvature)
  - abnormal lordosis (concave curvature)
  - scoliosis (curving away from the midline).

Curvature of a normal spine

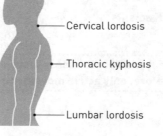

Cervical lordosis

Thoracic kyphosis

Lumbar lordosis

- Next, ask the patient to stand, back against the wall. Normally you should see the following in contact with the wall: occiput, shoulders, buttocks, heels. If not the spine is abnormal. Measures wall-occiput distance.

Palpation

Feel for the following bony landmarks:

- Vertebrae prominens at the C7/T1 junction
- Spinous processes from C6 to the sacrum
- Facet joints (that lie 1cm lateral to the spinous processes).
- Sacroiliac joints (beneath the dimples of Venus at S2).

Palpate the paraspinal muscles for tenderness (abnormal curvature can be due to muscle spasm).

Measure

Schober's test

- Identify the dimples of Venus (small depressions in the skin on either side of the midline around S2).
- Use a tape measure, and mark (with water-soluble ink) a point 10cm superior and 5cm inferior to the dimples.
- Ask the patient to touch their toes.
- The distance between the two marks should be measured at this stage, with the spine flexed.
- In a normal spine, the distance will increase to at least 21 cm.

Schober's test
(D = dimple of Venus)

Assess movements

> It is not possible to assess movements passively in the spine.
> Therefore, only active movements are tested.

Cervical spine

Test the following movements:

- Flexion (looking down at toes)

- Extension (looking up at ceiling)
- Lateral flexion (putting each ear onto the shoulder in turn)
- Lateral rotation (looking over each shoulder in turn).

Fix the shoulders when assessing flexion, to ensure that movement is occurring at the cervical spine rather than the shoulders.

Thoracic and lumbar spine

Test the following movements:

- Flexion (touching toes)
- Extension (leaning backwards)
- Lateral flexion (sliding the hand down the side of the right leg and then the left)
- Lateral rotation (twisting at the waist to the left and then the right).

Fix the pelvis when assessing lateral rotation. Do this by stabilising the pelvis with your hands, or performing the examination with the patient seated.

Special tests

Straight-leg raising test (for nerve root irritation)

With the patient supine, use your arm to fix the patient's pelvis across the anterior superior iliac spines. The patient then attempts to flex the hip as far as possible, with the knee fully extended (ie raise a straight leg towards the ceiling).

Stretch test (for sciatic nerve root irritation)

With the limit of straight-leg raising reached, allow the leg to lower slightly, then dorsiflex the foot (push the toes towards the head) quickly. If this causes severe pain the test is positive.

Test function

Ask the patient to:

- put on a coat
- take off and put on their shoes.

Thank the patient

Turn and face the examiner

Examiners' favourites

Q List some risk factors for primary osteoporosis.

A Female gender, postmenopausal status, small frame, lack of exercise, smoking, excess alcohol, family history, poor intake of dairy products.

Q List four extra-articular features of ankylosing spondylitis.

A Anterior uveitis, aortic regurgitation, pulmonary fibrosis, Achilles tendonitis.

Summary

ICE
▼
Inspect from the end of the bed
▼
Inspect the spine
▼
Palpate the spine
▼
Perform Schober's test
▼
Test active movements in the cervical spine
▼
Test active movements in the thoracic and lumbar spines
▼
Perform the straight-leg raising test
▼
Perform the stretch test
▼
Test function
▼
Thank the patient
▼
Turn and face the examiner

Hip pathology may present with knee pain as they share obturator and femoral nerve supply. For this reason, the hip should be examined in patients presenting with knee pain.

ICE

- Introduce yourself.
- Consent the patient for the examination.
- Expose the necessary parts of the body and position the patient. The whole lower limb should be exposed – ask the patient to remove any trousers but to keep underwear on. Use a blanket to preserve dignity. The patient should be standing initially.

Examination

Inspection

From the end of the bed

- Look around the bed for clues, eg walking stick, Delta Rollator, orthopaedic shoes.
- Scan the patient from head to toe, and note:
  - Does the patient look well or unwell?
  - Does the patient have any obvious conditions, eg a recent surgical scar?

Legs

With the patient standing

Inspect from in front, the side and behind. Look for:

- scars
- skin changes
- deformities
- muscle wasting
- swelling – bony or soft-tissue.

When inspecting from behind, look particularly at the level of the iliac crests and for the presence of a raised gluteal fold.

With the patient walking (if possible)
Look for:

- use of a walking aid
- abnormal gait pattern
- abnormal stride length
- evidence of pain.

With the patient on the bed
The angle of the bed should be 45°.

You will require full exposure of the pelvic region to inspect properly. You should look at both sides from in front and from behind (ie the buttocks).

Palpation

The patient should remain on the bed. Feel for the major landmarks:

- Anterior superior iliac spine (ASIS)
- Ischial spine.

In some circumstances it may be necessary to palpate for temperature and tenderness of the hip joint, but as it is a deep-seated joint, this is rarely of any value.

Measure

Use a measuring tape to measure:

- apparent length: xiphisternum to medial malleolus
- true length: ASIS to medial malleolus.

Some will advise that the umbilicus should be used as a landmark for measurement rather than the xiphisternum. The latter should be used since it is a fixed point.

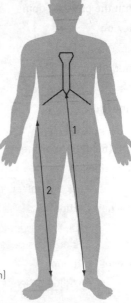

Measuring leg length
(1 = apparent length; 2 = true length)

Active movements

> The pelvis should be fixed when you are assessing movements of the hip. This is to ensure that the movement observed is due to movement of the hip joint and not the pelvis. The pelvis is fixed by using the left hand to stabilise the contralateral ASIS.

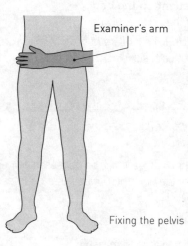

Examiner's arm

Fixing the pelvis

With the patient supine:

Flexion

Ask the patient to bring the heel up to the bottom.

Abduction

Ask the patient to move a straight leg away from the mid-line.

Adduction

Ask the patient to move a straight leg across the mid-line.

With the patient prone:

Extension

Ask the patient to lie prone, and to raise each leg off the bed.

Internal rotation

Ask the patient to keep the knees tight together, and spread the ankles as far apart as possible.

External rotation

Ask the patient to cross the legs over as shown in the diagram.

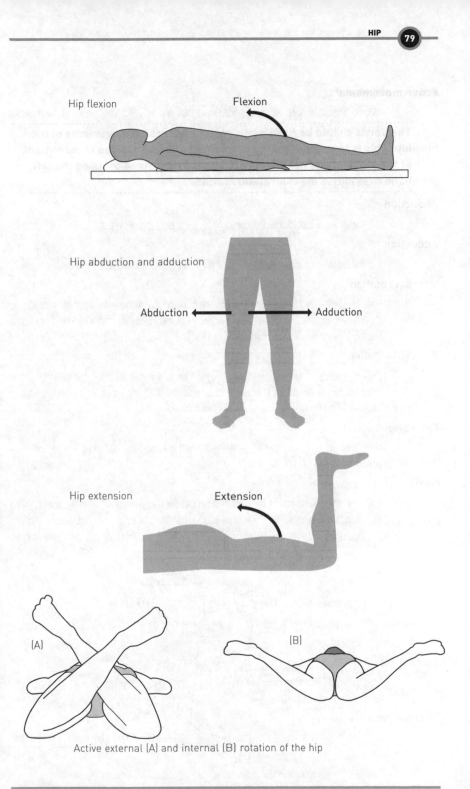

Hip flexion

Flexion

Hip abduction and adduction

Abduction ← → Adduction

Hip extension

Extension

(A)

(B)

Active external (A) and internal (B) rotation of the hip

Passive movements

Work through the above movements again. Perform the movements yourself, rather than asking the patient.

Flexion

Move the heel up towards the bottom (as with active) and then push the knee towards the patient's body.

Abduction

As for active, but done by examiner with patient relaxed.

Adduction

As for active, but done by examiner with patient relaxed.

Internal rotation

Flex the knee and stabilise it with one hand. With the other hand, move the heel laterally. The heel moves away from the midline, but the knee and hip rotate internally (ie towards the midline).

External rotation

Flex the knee and stabilise it with one hand. With the other hand, move the heel medially. The heel moves towards the midline, but the knee and hip rotate externally (ie away from the midline).

Extension

With the patient prone, lift the thigh up off the bed by pulling the foot directly upwards.

Internal and external rotation can also be tested with the hip extended. With the patient lying prone, flex the knee to 90°, and then move the feet to separate them (internal rotation) and to cross them over (external rotation).

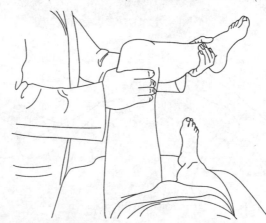

Passive external rotation of the hip

> **Be sure that you are not causing the patient any pain when testing passive movements.**

Special tests

Trendelenburg test

- Observe the patient from behind.

Ask them to support their weight on the right hip only (ie ask them to lift the left leg off the ground by bending the knee).

- Watch the pelvis, and note the direction of tilt. (In normal individuals, the pelvis will rise on the side of the leg that has been lifted. With instability, the pelvis may drop on the side of the leg that has been lifted.)
- Repeat the test, with the patient standing on the other leg.

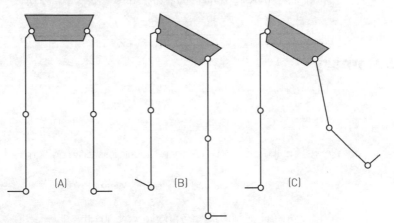

Trendelenburg test: (A) standing on both legs; (B) normal - the pelvis rises on the side of the lifted leg; (C) abnormal - the pelvis drops on the side of the lifted leg

Thomas' test

- Put your left hand (palm upwards) beneath the lumbar spine to ensure that the lumbar spine remains flattened during the test.
- With the other hand, passively flex one hip.
- While you are flexing this hip, observe the movement of the other leg – in the event of a fixed flexion deformity (common in hip osteoarthritis), the opposite leg flexes too.
- Repeat the test on the other hip.

Test function

Gait should have been assessed earlier in your examination.

Thank the patient

Turn and face the examiner

> **Examiner's favourites**
>
> **Q** What is the first movement to become affected in osteoarthritis of the hip?
>
> **A** Internal rotation of the hip.
>
> **Q** What are the four characteristic radiological features of osteoarthritis of the hip?
>
> **A** Loss of joint space, subchondral bone sclerosis, osteophyte formation and bony cyst formation.

Summary

ICE
▼
Inspect from the end of the bed
▼
Inspect the legs with the patient standing, walking and on the bed
▼
Palpate the hip joints
▼
Measure apparent leg length
▼
Measure true leg length
▼
Test active movements
▼
Test passive movements
▼
Perform the Trendelenburg test
▼
Perform Thomas' test
▼
Thank the patient
▼
Turn and face the examiner

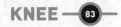

ICE

- Introduce yourself.
- Consent the patient for the examination.
- Expose the necessary parts of the body and position the patient. The whole lower limb should be exposed – ask the patient to remove any trousers, but to keep underwear on. Use a blanket to preserve dignity. The patient should be standing initially.

Examination

Inspection

From the end of the bed

- Look around the bed for clues, eg walking stick, Delta Rollator.
- Scan the patient from head to toe, and note:
  - Does the patient look well or unwell?
  - Does the patient have any obvious conditions, eg a recent surgical scar?

Legs

With the patient standing

Inspect the knees from in front, the side and from behind. Look for:

- scars
- skin changes
- deformities
- muscle wasting
- swelling – bony, soft-tissue or fluid.

With the patient walking (if possible)

Inspect the patient's gait as they to walk to the other side of the room, turn, and come back.

With the patient on the bed

The angle of the bed should be 45°. Inspect the knees close up for fine details such as scars, small volumes of fluid, cysts and muscle state.

Palpation

The patient should remain on the bed. Feel for:

- temperature (use the back of the hand to feel the temperature over the knee and compare sides)
- the quadriceps tendon, patella and patellar ligament

- the joint line (ask the patient to bend the knee slightly while doing this to confirm the location of the joint line)
- the collateral ligaments
- the patellofemoral joint, including beneath the patella.

Test for the presence of a joint effusion, using either the bulge test (if a little fluid is present) or the patellar tap test (for a larger volume of fluid).

Bulge test

Using the curve formed between your extended thumb and index finger, milk down any fluid from above the knee.

Using your index and middle fingers together as a unit, sweep any fluid along the medial aspect of the knee (see 1 in the diagram). Then sweep along the lateral side of the knee, and watch to see if a bulge occurs on the medial side (see 2 in the diagram).

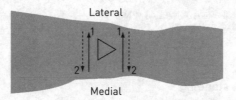

Bulge test (see text for legend to numbers)

Patellar tap test

1 Using the curve formed between the thumb and the index finger, milk down any fluid from above the knee.

2 Using the index and middle fingers of the other hand, push (not tap) the patella down firmly. If fluid is present the patella will bounce off the lateral femoral condyle behind. This makes a tapping noise – hence the name of the test.

Measure

Using a tape measure, obtain the circumference (in centimetres) of both legs around the bulk of the quadriceps muscles. Measure from a fixed bony point so that an identical position is used for both sides.

Active movements

Flexion

Ask the patient to bend their knee.

Extension

Ask the patient to straighten their leg.

Passive movements

Work through the movements again. Perform the movements yourself, rather than asking the patient to perform them.

Flexion

Bend the leg at the knee.

Extension

Straighten the leg at the knee. Place your hand over the patella while doing this, and feel for crepitus.

Hyperextension

- Lift the leg off the bed and gently push the knee downwards from above to see if it will extend further.
- Lifting the leg off the couch also allows one to look for tibial sag (which is seen when the posterior cruciate ligament is damaged).

Be sure that you are not causing the patient any pain when testing passive movements.

Special tests

Test the integrity of the collateral ligaments

Flex the knee to 30°. Support the medial aspect of the thigh, and push medially on the lower leg (shown in bold in the diagram below). This tests the lateral collateral ligament. Then, support the lateral aspect of the thigh, and push laterally on the lower leg (shown in capital letters in the diagram below). This tests the medial collateral ligament. Excessive movement indicates ligament damage.

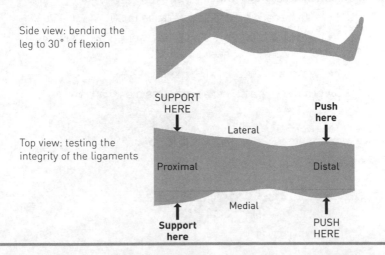

Side view: bending the leg to 30° of flexion

Top view: testing the integrity of the ligaments

SUPPORT HERE

Push here

Lateral

Proximal

Distal

Medial

Support here

PUSH HERE

Test the integrity of the cruciate ligaments

The integrity of these ligaments may be assessed using the anterior and posterior drawer tests (which are performed at the same time). With both tests it is essential that the patient is relaxed.

- With the patient supine on the couch, ask them to flex their knee to about 100°.

- Palpate the bulk of the quadriceps muscles to ensure that the patient is relaxed.

- After checking that there is no pain in the foot, perch yourself (one buttock) on the foot to stabilise the lower leg.

- With both hands, wrap your fingers around the back of the knee, keeping the thumbs in front over the patella. Position the thumbs so they point directly towards the ceiling.

- Pull/push the unit you have formed with your hands forward (to test anterior cruciate) and backwards (to test posterior cruciate).

Excessive movement indicates ligament damage.

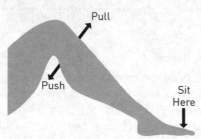

Position of leg for testing the cruciate ligaments. Pulling tests the anterior ligament; pushing tests the posterior ligament.

Testing the menisci (Apley's grinding test)

- With the patient prone, flex the knee to 90°.

- Use your left hand to stabilise the lower leg behind the knee and with the right hand grip the heel of the foot.

- Twist the foot in a 'grinding motion'.

A grinding sensation or pain indicates meniscal damage.

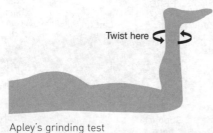

Apley's grinding test

Examine the hips

The knee and hip share a partially similar nerve supply. The knee is therefore an important source of referred hip pain, especially in children. Therefore, all knee examinations should be accompanied by a hip examination. If time limitations in an examination do not permit this, you should state that it would be your intention to examine the hip as well.

Thank the patient

Turn and face the examiner

Examiner's favourites

Q What are the common causes of a palpable mass behind the knee?

A Sebaceous cyst, popliteal artery aneurysm, semimembranosus bursa, Baker's cyst.

Q Outline the treatment options for osteoarthritis of the knee.

A Analgesia, physiotherapy, wedge tibial osteotomy, total joint replacement.

Summary

ICE

▼

Inspect from the end of the bed

▼

Inspect the legs with the patient standing, walking and on the bed

▼

Palpate the knee joints

▼

Test for a joint effusion

▼

Measure quadriceps bulk

▼

Test active movements

▼

Test passive movements

▼

▼

Test the integrity of the collateral ligaments

▼

Test the integrity of the cruciate ligaments

▼

Test the integrity of the menisci

▼

Examine the hips

▼

Thank the patient

▼

Turn and face the examiner

ICE

- Introduce yourself.
- Consent the patient for the examination.
- Expose the necessary parts of the body and position the patient. The whole lower limb should be exposed – ask the patient to remove any trousers but to keep underwear on. Use a blanket to preserve the patient's dignity. The patient should be standing initially.

Examination

Inspection

From the end of the bed

- Look around the bed for clues, eg walking stick, Delta Rollator, orthopaedic shoe.
- Scan the patient from head to toe, and note:
  - Does the patient look well or unwell?
  - Does the patient have any obvious conditions, eg a recent surgical scar?

> Be attentive to the nature of their footwear and how the shoe has worn. The back of the shoe may reveal wear suggestive of abnormal loading.

Legs

With the patient standing

Inspect the ankles and feet from in front, the side and behind. Look for:

- scars
- skin changes
- deformities
- muscle wasting
- swelling – bony, soft-tissue or fluid
- foot arches (longitudinal and transverse); pes cavus (high arched foot) or pes plantus (flat foot)
- ulcers.

With the patient walking (if possible)

Inspect the patient's gait as they walk to the other side of the room, turn, and come back. Observe first with the patient wearing footwear, then barefoot (as shoes may hide some abnormalities).

With the patient on the bed

The angle of the bed should be 45°.

- Inspect the ankles and feet close up for fine details, such as scars, callosities or ulcers.
- Inspect the toes for ingrowing toenails, atrophic toenails, mallet toe, hammer toe (usually 2nd toe), bunion (1st metatarso–phalangeal [MTP] joint), bunionette (5th MTP joint) or clawing.

Palpation

The patient should remain on the bed. Feel for:

- temperature – feel over the main joints with the dorsum of your hand
- bony prominences – lateral/medial malleoli, MTP joints, interphalangeal (IP) joints and heel; squeeze across metatarsal joints (as shown in the diagram) and note any pain

Squeezing across the metatarsal joints

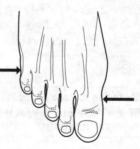

- Achilles' tendon – feel for a palpable gap in the tendon indicating a rupture
- spurs – press deep into the sole of the foot to feel for spurs.

Measure

Measure the 'calf girth' on both sides, in order to obtain an objective measure of any muscle wasting or hypertrophy.

Active movements

Movements take place at the ankle joint, subtarsal joint, mid-tarsal joint, MTP and IP joints. Movements should be performed while the patient is sitting on the edge of the bed, with the legs hanging over the edge (knees flexed and lower leg relaxed).

Dorsiflexion

Ask the patient to point the toes towards their head.

Plantar flexion

Ask the patient to point the toes towards the floor.

Inversion

Fix the calcaneum with your hand, and ask the patient to turn the sole in towards the midline.

Eversion

Fix the calcaneum with your hand, and ask the patient to turn the sole away from the midline.

Toe flexion

Ask the patient to curl their toes.

Toe extension

Ask the patient to straighten their toes.

Toe abduction

Ask the patient to fan the toes.

Toe adduction

Ask the patient to try to hold a piece of paper between the toes.

Passive movements

Work through the movements again. Perform the movements yourself, rather than asking the patient to perform them.

> **Be sure that you are not causing the patient any pain when you are testing passive movements.**

Special tests (if indicated)

Simmond's (squeeze) test (to test for rupture of the Achilles' tendon)

Ask the patient to kneel on a chair with their feet hanging over the edge, holding the back of the chair for steadiness. Squeeze the gastrocnemius muscle gently. Normally, the foot will plantar-flex. If the Achilles tendon is ruptured, no plantar flexion will occur.

Thank the patient

Turn and face the examiner

Examiners' favourites

Q Which muscles dorsiflex the foot?

A Tibialis anterior, extensor hallucis longus, extensor digitorum longus, peroneus tertius.

Q What clinical features are present in a common peroneal nerve injury?

A Foot drop, foot inversion and loss of sensation on the anterolateral surface of the leg and foot.

Summary

ICE
▼
Inspect from the end of the bed
▼
Inspect the legs with the patient standing, walking, and sitting on the bed
▼
Palpate the ankles and feet
▼
Measure calf girth
▼
Test active movements
▼
Test passive movements
▼
Thank the patient
▼
Turn and face the examiner

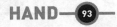

This chapter details the full examination of the hand. It should be read in conjunction with the chapter on hand joints and wrist (see page 57).

ICE

- Introduce yourself
- Consent the patient for the examination
- Expose the necessary parts of the body and position the patient. Roll the patient's sleeves up to the elbow, and place the hands on a white pillow. The patient can be seated for this examination.

Examination

Inspection

From the end of the bed

- Look around the bed for clues, eg occupational therapy aids for holding cups and unscrewing lids.
- Scan the patient from head to toe, and note:
  - Do they look well or unwell?
  - Do they have any obvious conditions, eg myotonic dystrophy?

Inspect the hands

Inspect the dorsal surfaces. Look for:

- nail abnormalities
- skin changes
- obvious joint deformity
- muscle wasting.

Inspect the palmar surfaces. Look for:

- skin changes, eg Dupuytren's contracture, palmar erythema
- muscle wasting
- abnormalities in the palmar creases eg pallor, pigmentation.

Inspect the outstretched hands from the side. Look for:

- finger drop
- tremor.

Palpation

Note the temperature of the hands. Examine the hand joints as detailed on page 58.

Palpate any abnormalities identified on inspection.

Movement

Test active and passive movements in all the hand joints. See pages 59-61 for details.

Test for the presence of myotonia by asking the patient to make a fist and then open it quickly. A patient with myotonia will not be able to perform this action quickly.

Test sensation

Test the modalities of light touch, pain, vibration sense and joint position sense in both peripheral nerve and dermatome distributions. See page 44 for further details. Peripheral nerve distributions are tested as follows:

- Radial nerve: touch in the anatomical snuffbox on the dorsal aspect.
- Ulnar nerve: touch over the medial one and a half fingers on the palm (little finger, and medial half of ring finger).
- Median nerve: touch over the lateral three and a half fingers on the palm (lateral half of ring finger, middle finger, index finger and thumb).

Assess pulses

Palpate the radial and ulnar pulses. You may also wish to perform Allan's test of perfusion of the hand.

Allan's Test

- Ask the patient to make a fist.
- Occlude both the radial and ulnar arteries by pressing over them.
- Press for 5 seconds.
- Ask the patient to open the palm and release the pressure on each artery in turn and watch the colour of the palm.
- It should change from pale to pink as blood flow is re-established.

Examine the elbows

In particular, look for rheumatoid nodules and the skin changes of psoriasis.

Test function

Ask the patient to:

- write their name
- fasten and undo a button
- pour and drink a glass of water.

Special tests (optional)

Perform Tinel's and Phalen's test as detailed on page 62.

Test for Froment's sign

To do this, ask the patient to hold a piece of paper/card between the thumbs and the radial aspect of the index finger. Then pull the paper away and ask the patient to stop it. With paralysis of adductor pollicis, the thumb will flex at the interphalangeal joint.

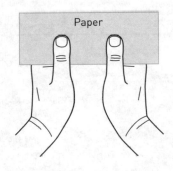

Perform Finklestein's test

Ask the patient to flex their thumb. Now, ulnar deviate the wrist. Pain is indicative of De Quervain's tenosynovitis.

Thank the patient

Turn and face the examiner

Examiners' Favourites

Q Name six signs of liver disease in the hands.

A Leuconychia, finger clubbing, palmar erythema, Dupuytren's contracture, spider naevi, xanthomata.

Q What nail changes may be present in a patient with psoriasis?

A Pitting, onycholysis, grease spots.

Summary

ICE
▼
Inspect from the end of the bed
▼
Inspect the hands
▼
Palpate the hands
▼
Test active movements at the wrist, thumb and fingers
▼
Test passive movements at the wrist, thumb and fingers
▼
Test for myotonia
▼
Test sensation
▼
Assess pulses
▼
Examine the elbows
▼
Test function
▼
Perform Tinel's test
▼
Perform Phalen's test
▼
Test for Froment's sign (optional)
▼
Perform Finklestein's test (optional)
▼
Thank the patient
▼
Turn and face the examiner

ICE

- **I**ntroduce yourself.
- **C**onsent the patient for the examination.
- **E**xpose the necessary parts of the body and position the patient. The patient should sit opposite you in a chair or a bed. Remove any hearing aids if present.

Examination

Inspection

From the end of the bed

- Look around the bed for clues, eg a hearing aid.
- Scan the patient from head to toe, and note:
  - Does the patient look well or unwell?
  - Does the patient have any obvious conditions, eg the typical skull of Paget's disease?
  - Does the patient have any clues to disease of the ears that are immediately apparent, eg prostheses?

Ears

Inspect the external ear. Look for:

- scars – a postauricular scar usually indicates mastoid surgery, whereas an endaural scar usually indicates middle ear surgery
- skin lesions on the skin of the pinna and external auditory meatus, eg gouty tophi, otitis externa.

Palpate the ear and surrounding structures

- Pull gently on the pinna and ask the patient if the movement caused pain.
- Palpate for cervical lymphadenopathy. Check the parotid, pre- and posterior auricular nodes (see cervical lymph nodes examination).

Examine the ear canal and tympanic membrane

- Fit a suitably sized speculum (largest feasible) to an auroscope. Before inserting this instrument into the external auditory meatus, it is necessary to straighten the ear canal by pulling on the pinna gently. In adults, the pinna should be pulled posterosuperiorly, whereas in children, it should be pulled posteroinferiorly as shown in the diagram (overleaf).

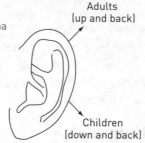

Direction to gently pull the pinna
to straighten the ear canal

Adults
(up and back)

Children
(down and back)

- The auroscope should be held like a pen, and the little finger of the hand holding the device should be extended. When the auroscope is inserted into the ear, the little finger should rest on the patient's cheek. This way, if the patient moves their head towards you, your whole hand is also moved, thus preventing the auroscope from entering too far into the ear canal.

- Slowly insert the auroscope, looking at the skin of the ear canal while it is going in. Inspect the tympanic membrane. Look at its appearance and position. Examine the attic, and look in the posterosuperior canal wall for an open mastoid cavity. Slowly retract the auroscope from the ear.

Test the hearing

Whisper test

This is a simple test designed to screen for hearing problems.

- Ask the patient to rub the external auditory canal of one ear with their finger while you test the other ear.

- Stand about 60 cm away from the patient, out of their line of vision and whisper a number. Whisper at the end of your breath to try to give a repeatable test. Good numbers to use are 100 and 68 since these assess a range of frequencies.

- Ask the patient to repeat this number.

- Repeat the test on the other ear.

Rinné's test

To interpret Rinné's and Weber's tests you have to understand that a healthy ear can hear sounds transmitted in the air better than those conducted by bone. This is because the ossicles in the middle ear amplify sound waves in the air.

- Strike a 512Hz tuning fork. Place the handle end of the fork on the patient's mastoid process. Then move it so that the vibrating part is adjacent to the ear canal.
- Ask the patient at which point the noise was louder. If the patient is unable to decide which was louder, the fork should be struck again. It is again held against the mastoid process, but this time the patient is asked to inform the doctor of the point when they can no longer hear the tone.
- At this moment, the tuning fork is moved in front of the ear canal, and the patient asked if they can again hear the tone.

Main parts of a tuning fork

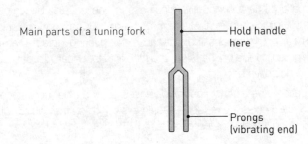

Hold handle here

Prongs (vibrating end)

If the patient has normal hearing, they should hear the tone loudest when the tuning fork is placed next to the ear canal. If they are unable to tell which tone is loudest, during the second test the tone will 'reappear' when the tuning fork is moved beside the ear canal. This is known as 'Rinné-positive' (normal).

However, patients with partial sensorineural (nerve) deafness will also be Rinné-positive. This is because all sounds are conducted to the brain via nerves, and if these nerves are damaged, both air and bone conduction are reduced.

If the patient has conductive deafness, the amplification system in the middle ear is defective. This means that the tone is heard loudest when the tuning fork is against the mastoid process. This is known as a 'Rinné-negative'.

Problems can arise if a patient has complete unilateral sensorineural hearing loss. You would expect that both air and bone conduction would be wiped out with this problem. However, a patient with this condition will be able to hear the tuning fork when it is placed on the mastoid process, but will not be able to hear it at all when it is placed at the ear canal. This is because with bone conduction the sound is conducted to the other ear, where it is heard. So the patient in this instance will produce a Rinné-negative result. However, since there is no conductive deafness, this is known as a 'false-negative Rinné'.

In order to distinguish between a true and false Rinné, the following test can be carried out.

Weber's test

A similar tuning fork to that used above is again struck. The base of the fork is placed in the centre of the forehead. The patient is asked to inform the doctor if the sound is heard equally in the two ears, or whether it is louder in one.

In normal subjects, the sound is conducted by the bone to both ears where it is heard equally.

If a patient has a conductive deafness in one ear, the background noise normally picked up by that ear is not heard. Bone conduction is equal in both ears. This means that, because the hearing defect masks out the background noise on that side, the tone is in fact heard loudest on the side of the defective ear.

If a patient has a sensorineural deafness on one side, both air- and bone-conducted noise are reduced. So, in this condition the sound will be heard loudest on the side of the good ear.

Summary of results in Rinné s and Weber's tests

Result	Rinné	Weber - loudest in:
Normal hearing	+ve	Both ears
Left conductive deafness	-ve	Left ear
Left partial sensorineural deafness	+ve	Right ear
Left complete sensorineural deafness	-ve	Right ear

Thank the patient

Turn and face the examiner

Examiners' favourites

Q Name three causes of conduction deafness.

A Wax, otosclerosis, otitis media.

Q Name three causes of sensorineural deafness.

A Acoustic neuroma, presbyacusis, aminoglycoside toxicity.

Summary

ICE

▼

Inspect from the end of the bed

▼

Inspect the ears

▼

Palpate the ears

▼

Palpate for cervical lymphadenopathy

▼

Examine the ear canal and tympanic membrane with an auroscope

▼

Perform the whisper test

▼

Perform Rinné's test

▼

Perform Weber's test

▼

Thank the patient

▼

Turn and face the examiner

Look for specific signs in the eye when you are performing an examination of a patient's body system. For example, examine the sclera for jaundice when you are examining the alimentary system. However, you should also be able to examine the eye in isolation. Individual components of the complete examination may be undertaken alone when indicated.

ICE

- Introduce yourself.
- Consent the patient for the examination.
- Expose the necessary parts of body and position the patient. The patient should be sitting opposite you on a chair.

Examination

Inspection

From the end of the bed

- Look around the bed for clues, eg spectacles, low vision aids, 'white stick'.
- Scan the patient from head to toe, and note:
  - Does the patient look well or unwell?
  - Does the patient have any apparent conditions, eg oculocutaneous albinism or myasthemia gravis?
  - Does the patient have any clues to eye disease that are immediately apparent, eg glass eye, proptosis?

Eyes

Look for:

- contact lenses
- redness and its distribution
- pupil size, shape and equality between sides
- abnormal positioning of the eyes
- proptosis (protrusion of the eye) – stand behind the patient and look over the top of their head to assess this
- strabismus (squint).

Eyelids

Look at the positions of the lids for ptosis (drooping), retraction or other abnormalities, eg ectropion (turning out) or entropion (turning in).

Eyebrows

Look for any abnormalities, eg thinning of the outer third may be seen in hypothyroidism.

Test visual acuity
Distance vision

> A standard Snellen chart should be read from a distance of 6 m (although in small rooms the chart is usually 3 m away from the patient with a mirror being used to effectively double this distance).

- Test each eye in turn by asking the patient to cover the eye not being tested. Spectacles or contact lenses should be worn. If the patient has forgotten their lenses, perform the test while the patient is looking through a pin hole.
- Start at the top of the chart (largest letters). Point to a row and ask the patient to identify the letters. Record the minimum size of print that the patient can see with each eye.

Record visual acuity in a standard fashion. For example, an acuity of 6/12 indicates that the patient can read letters from a distance of 6 m that a patient with perfect eyesight would be able to read at 12 m. (NB. There is normally a small number printed next to the row of letters being tested indicating the distance at which a patient with perfect visual acuity could read the letters.)

Smaller Snellen charts are available to assess visual acuity from the end of the bed.

Near vision
This test is carried out in much the same fashion as the Snellen chart test. Give the patient variously sized pieces of text, with the aim of recording the smallest sized text that they can read.

Colour vision
Give the patient pictures of numbers made up of various colours (Ishihara pseudoisochromatic plates). Ask the patient to identify what number is contained in the patterns. The aim of this test is to identify colour blindness.

Pupillary responses
Response to light

- Rest the ulnar aspect of your hand on the patient's nose to stop light being shone into both eyes.
- Ask the patient to focus on an object in the distance. Look at the size of the right pupil.

- Shine light from a pen torch into the right eye and watch for pupil constriction (direct response).
- Repeat this procedure for the left eye.
- Next, look at the left pupil, while shining the light into the right pupil. This should constrict again (consensual response).
- Finally, watch the right pupil while you shine the light into the left eye.

Response to accommodation

- While the patient is focusing on an object in the distance, place your index finger close to the patient (approximately 10 cm away), midway between the eyes. Watch the size of the right pupil as you ask the patient to shift their point of focus to your finger. The pupil should constrict.
- Repeat this again watching for constriction in the left pupil.

Test extraocular movements

> **Stabilise the patient's head with one of your hands (to ensure that it is the eyes that are moving, not the head).**

- Hold up one finger directly in front of the patient, about 50 cm away from the patient's face. Ask the patient to follow your finger with their eyes as you move through the main positions of gaze.

In order that all positions are tested, the following system may be helpful:

- Move your hand through the shape of the letter 'H'. This will test horizontal movement, as well as up and down gaze to the left and right.
- Next, return to the centre, and move your hand through the shape of the letter 'X'. This will test diagonal movement of the eyes in all positions.
- Finally, return to the centre again, and trace the shape of the letter 'I' (ie vertically up and down). Have the patient look upwards first to move to a downwards gaze slowly. As well as watching the eye movements here, look at the movement of the upper eyelid. It should drop down at approximately the same speed as the eye (lid lag is present if the lid movement lags behind the eye movement – this is seen with some thyroid disorders).

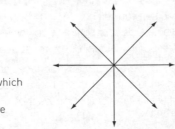

Directions in which
extraocular
movements are
assessed

Ask the patient if double vision (diplopia) was noticed in any of the
directions of gaze.

Assess visual fields

Visual fields may be tested using confrontation. On paper, the technique for
confrontation seems a little laborious. However, in practice, once this is
mastered, it can be performed very efficiently.

The seating arrangements of examiner and patient are crucial if visual
fields are to be assessed adequately.

- Sit on a chair directly opposite the seated patient about 1 m from the
  patient, so that your eyes are level with the patient's. The aim is to make
  movements with your hands that the patient is asked to identify, in order
  to assess whether the patient's visual fields are comparable to yours
  (assumed to be normal). It is vital that your hands are held midway
  between yourself and the patient.

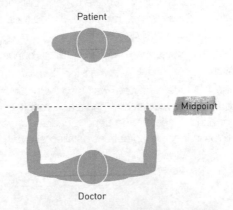

Patient

Midpoint

Doctor

Seating arrangements for confrontation (viewed from above)

- Place your arms as shown in the diagram. Reach your left arm upwards so that you can see your left hand in the upper temporal (lateral) quadrant of your left eye. Reach your right arm downwards so that you can see it in the lower temporal quadrant of your right eye.

- Ask the patient to look directly at your nose, and to close one eye. You (the examiner) should look at the patient's nose and close the opposite eye to the patient (ie if the patient closes their right eye, you should close your left eye).

- Encourage the patient to concentrate on looking at your nose for the duration of the examination and not to be tempted to look at your hands.

- Inform the patient that you are going to be moving the fingers of either your left or right hand. Ask the patient to identify (by pointing or otherwise) on which hand the fingers are being moved. The aim is to move your hands inwards from the periphery so that you can just see the fingers of the hand moving. When your hand is at this point, it is at the edge of your visual field. To do this, bring your left hand very slowly downwards and towards the nose (always keeping the hand at an equal distance between you and the patient). Wiggle your index finger and stop moving your hand when you can just see your finger moving. If the patient's visual fields are identical to yours, he or she should also be able to see your fingers at this point. If not, continue to move your hand downwards and towards the nose until the movement has been noticed. Assess whether or not the limit of the patient's visual field is significantly different from yours.

- Next, move your right hand in a similar manner. This time, move upwards and towards the nose. Note the point at which you can see your finger moving, and compare this to that reported by the patient.

- Repeat these movements several times, alternating on which of the hands the finger is wiggled. Ensure that the patient can correctly identify on which hand the finger is being moved, and try to accurately determine the limits of these visual quadrants.

- Occasionally, move the fingers on both hands (to test for visual inattention).

- Next, reach your left arm downwards so that your left hand is seen in the lower quadrant of your left eye, and reach your right arm upwards so that the right hand is seen in the upper quadrant of your right eye. Assess visual fields in these quadrants as detailed above.

- Once all four quadrants have been tested, you should examine for a central scotoma (blind area). A hat pin with a red head is commonly used for this. This should be held laterally, and slowly moved in the midline (ie between upper and lower fields) towards the nose. The patient should be asked to identify any regions in which they are unable to see the red part of the pin. (NB. A small 'blind spot' is present in all individuals, but this area can be much larger with certain eye problems.) The patient must again look at your nose for this test.
- Once these tests are complete, both patient and examiner should switch eyes and assess the visual fields in the other eye.

Perform fundoscopy

Warn the patient that you will get very close to their face during the examination, and also that the light from the ophthalmoscope is quite bright.

The patient should remove any spectacles.

If possible, switch the ophthalmoscope light beam to a large circle, to enable optimal viewing.

- Fundoscopy is much easier if the pupil has been dilated with a mydriatic drug, such as tropicamide.
- To examine the patient's right eye, hold the direct ophthalmoscope in your right hand, and look through it with your right eye. Similarly, use your left side to examine the patient's left eye.
- Ask the patient to look straight ahead. Stand about 1 m away from the patient, and look through the ophthalmoscope at the eye. The red reflex should be visible (ie the pupil should appear red). Focus the instrument to give a clear image. While still looking through the device, move closer to the patient, until the ophthalmoscope is close to the eye (2–3 cm away). Reach out with the hand not holding the ophthalmoscope, and gently support the patient's upper eyelid in the open position (so that blinking does not obstruct your examination).
- Once you are close to the patient, use the focus control on the ophthalmoscope to obtain a sharp image of the fundus. Identify a blood vessel, and follow its course (as it gets bigger) until you can see the optic disc. Note the following features of the optic disc: size; colour; cup:disc ratio; margins (distinct or blurred).
- Follow each of the major blood vessels along its course, starting at the optic disc. Note the features listed in the box.

Features of retinal blood vessels (the 4 Cs)

- Colour (eg normal, orange, white)
- Calibre (eg normal, narrowed)
- Course (eg undulating, tortuous)
- Crossing of arterioles and veins (note the angle of crossing, and whether or not the vein appears to be nipped by the arteriole)

- Next, scan the retina in all four quadrants and note any abnormalities. Ask the patient to look directly at the light, to allow assesment of the macula.
- Repeat on the other eye.

Slit lamp examination (if available)

The slit lamp is used primarily for examining the anterior segment of the eye.

- Ask the patient to place the chin on the chin rest, and the forehead on the support. Adjust the light beam so that a ray of light is evident on the patient's eye.
- Look through the eyepieces. Adjust the lamp until you can see a focused image. Select an appropriate beam of light for what you are examining, eg use a wide beam for scanning large areas, and a narrow beam for examining smaller details.
- Angle the beam of light obliquely across the cornea to estimate the corneal thickness.
- Closely inspect aspects of the eye nearest the outside (eyelids, eyelashes etc) and work your way inwards towards the anterior vitreous.
- Test the pupillary reaction to light and also the red reflex.

Perform the cover/uncover test (when applicable)

V This tests for a manifest squint.

- Ask the patient to focus on an object held about 30 cm from the eyes.
- Watch the right eye carefully, and cover up the left eye (eg with a piece of card). If the right eye moves, the patient has a 'manifest squint'. The type of squint depends on the direction in which the eye moves:
  - lateral movement (ie the eye turns outwards) = convergent squint
  - medial movement (ie the eye turns inwards) = divergent squint
  - upward movement = hypotropia;
  - downward movement = hypertropia.
- Remove the cover from the left eye. Watch the left eye carefully, and note any movement in it as you cover the right eye.
- Repeat the test with the patient focusing at an object 6 m away.

V If no squint is observed, the alternate cover test should be performed.

Alternate cover test

V This tests for a latent squint.

- Quickly cover the left and right eyes alternately several times in succession.
- Then cover the right eye for a few seconds.
- Remove the cover and watch the right eye closely as the cover is removed. If the right eye moves, the patient has a 'latent squint'. The type of squint depends on the direction in which the eye moves:
  - lateral movement = esophoria
  - medial movement = exophoria
  - upward movement = hypophoria;
  - downward movement = hyperphoria.
- This procedure can then be repeated, covering and watching the left eye.

Thank the patient

Turn and face the examiner

Examiners' favourites

Q List some causes of an absent red reflex.

A Glass eye, corneal opacity, cataract, vitreous haemorrhage, retinal detachment.

Q List three causes of a bitemporal hemianopia.

A Pituitary tumour, craniopharyngioma, suprasellar meningioma.

Summary

ICE
▼
Inspect from the end of the bed
▼
Inspect the eyes
▼
Inspect the eyelids
▼
Inspect the eyebrows
▼
Test visual acuity (distance and near) and colour vision
▼
Test pupillary responses to light and accommodation
▼
Test extraocular movements
▼
Assess visual fields
▼
Perform fundoscopy
▼
Perform a slit lamp examination (if available)
▼
Perform the cover/uncover test (if applicable)
▼
Perform the alternate cover test (if applicable)
▼
Thank the patient
▼
Turn and face the examiner

It is of paramount importance in examining the breast of any patient that you show dignity and respect for what is one of the most private parts of the body.

The breast examination should be part of the complete examination of a female patient.

ICE

- Introduce yourself.
- Consent the patient for the examination.
- Expose the necessary parts of the body and position the patient. Ask her to remove any tops and her brassiere. Cover her with a blanket when you are not examining the breasts. Position the back of the bed at 45° to the horizontal.

Examination

A female chaperone should always be present for this examination.

Inspection

From the end of the bed

- Look around the bed for signs of other illnesses.
- Scan the patient from head to toe, and note:
  - Does the patient look well or unwell?
  - Does the patient have any obvious conditions?
  - What is her body habitus, eg normal weight, cachectic?
  - What is the patient's colour, eg pale, cyanosed, jaundiced, ruddy complexion?

Breasts

Examine both breasts on all occasions, starting with the normal breast if an abnormality is known to be on one side.

Inspect with the patient in three different positions (as shown in the diagram overleaf). The positions tense various muscle groups, helping to accentuate the surface features of breast pathology.

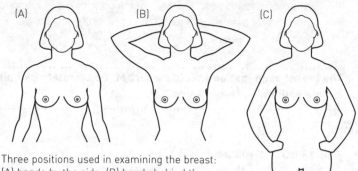

Three positions used in examining the breast:
(A) hands by the side; (B) hands behind the
head; (C) hands on the hips

Look for:

- pitting
- peau d'orange (resembles the dimpled skin of an orange)
- puckering
- tethering
- prominent veins
- scars or candidiasis in the sub-mammary folds
- scars from previous procedures or radiotherapy
- the five 'D's of the nipple:
    - discharge
    - discoloration
    - dermatological change, eg Paget's disease (appearance of eczema around the nipple)
    - depression or in-drawing
    - deviation.

Palpation

Breasts

Ask if there is any pain in the breasts before palpating

Bear in mind that a breast may have been reconstructed or contain an implant.

Palpate for masses

Use the path shown in the diagram to guide your examination.

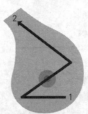

Path taken during examination of the breast. 1 = start point; 2 = end point

If a lump is noted, describe it using the following scheme:

Characterisation of a breast lump (3 Ss, 3 Cs, 3 Ts)		
• Site	• Colour	• Tethering
• Size	• Contour	• Transillumination
• Shape	• Consistency	• Temperature

Palpation should be done with smooth, circular, flowing movements of the finger-tips. This allows the breast to be rolled between the fingers and the underlying chest wall. Be firm, but gentle, to identify any lumps.

Make sure that you palpate the axillary tail.

• Palpate the nipple, and gently squeeze to assess for discharge.

Inspect the axillae

Support the patient's arm, and inspect on both sides for visible lumps or skin changes.

Palpate the axillae

Stand behind the patient when you are palpating the axillae.

• Support the patient's arm, and palpate all five walls of the axillae: medial, lateral, anterior, posterior and apex (roof).

Palpate for supra-clavicular lymph nodes (see cervical lymph nodes examination)

Palpate the liver (see alimentary system examination)

Palpation of the liver is necessary in order to detect metastatic deposits. If these are extensive, the liver may be hard, craggy and irregular.

Examine the chest (see respiratory system examination)

Examine the chest for the presence of a malignant pleural effusion. If present, this is likely to be unilateral.

Palpate the spine

Examine the spine for tenderness that may result from bony metastases.

Thank the patient

Cover the patient

Turn and face the examiner

Examiners' favourites

Q Which group of patients are currently called for breast cancer screening?

A All women aged between 50 and 65 are currently called for 3-yearly screening mammography. It is likely in the near future that the upper-end range will be extended to 70 years of age.

Q What is meant by the triple assessment of breast lumps?

A This relates to the three-stage approach carried out at many breast clinics: clinical examination, imaging and histological assessment.

Summary

ICE
▼
Inspect from the end of the bed
▼
Inspect the breasts
▼
Palpate the breasts
▼
Inspect the axillae
▼
Palpate the axillae
▼
Palpate for supraclavicular lymph nodes
▼
Palpate the liver
▼
Examine the chest
▼
Palpate the spine
▼
Thank the patient
▼
Cover the patient
▼
Turn and face the examiner

You may be asked to examine the cervical lymph nodes on their own, but it is more likely that you will use this examination as part of a more thorough systems evaluation, such as the respiratory system.

ICE

- **I**ntroduce yourself.
- **C**onsent the patient for the examination.
- **E**xpose the necessary parts of the body and position the patient. The neck should be well exposed. This examination is best carried out by standing behind the seated patient.

Examination

Inspection

From the end of the bed

- Look around the bed for clues, eg dietary requirements for patients with swallowing problems.
- Scan the patient from head to toe, and note:
  - Does the patient look well or unwell?
  - Does the patient have any obvious conditions, eg large parotid tumour?
  - What is the patient's colour, eg pale, cyanosed, jaundiced?

Palpation

Some doctors advise that both sides should be examined simultaneously; others prefer to examine each side in isolation.

There are two chains of nodes: circular and vertical. The examination begins with the circular chain.

Examination of the circular chain of lymph nodes

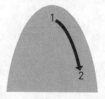 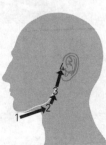 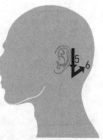

(A) The underside of the patient's chin and mandible–submental (point 1) and submandibular (point 2) nodes

(B) Parotid nodes (point 3) and pre-auricular node (point 4)

(C) Posterior auricular (point 5) and occipital nodes nodes (point 6)

The first diagram (A) represents the underside of the patient's chin and mandible.

- Begin at the point marked 1 (submental nodes), feel for any abnormalities with the flats of your fingers, moving in a circular motion.

- Work your way round to point 2, which is at the angle of the mandible. The submandibular nodes lie at this point.

- Without lifting your fingers off the patient's face, work your way to point 3 as shown the second diagram (B). This is the location of the parotid nodes.

- Continue towards point 4. This point is directly anterior to the tragus of the ear and is the position of the pre-auricular node.

- Next, move your fingers to the posterior side of the ear pinna, and feel for the posterior auricular nodes – point 5 in the third diagram (C).

- When you have examined the inferior aspect of the mastoid process, move on to the posterior aspect of the head and palpate for the occipital nodes (point 6).

This completes the examination of the circular chain of lymph nodes.

Next, the vertical chain of lymph nodes must be examined:

Examination of the vertical chain of lymph nodes. Sternomastoid muscle (point 7); scalene node (point 8); supraclavicular fossa (point 9); posterior triangle of the neck (point 10)

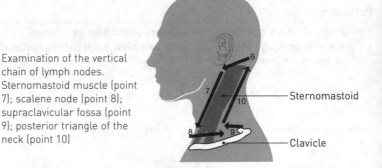

- Ask the patient to relax their shoulders. Work your way along the anterior border of the sternomastoid muscle (point 7).

- At its inferior end, palpate the muscle between finger and thumb to feel for the scalene node (point 8).

- Next, move laterally and examine the supraclavicular fossa (point 9).

- Finally, work your way up towards the occipital region again, by palpating the posterior border of the sternomastoid muscle and the posterior triangle of the neck (point 10).

If lymphadenopathy is detected, it may be appropriate to examine other lymph node areas. These include the axillary, epitrochlear (at the elbow), inguinal and popliteal nodes. The liver and spleen should also be palpated for enlargement.

Thank the patient

Turn and face the examiner

Examiners' favourites

Q List two causes of occipital lymphadenopathy.

A Head lice, rubella infection.

Q What is Troisier's sign?

A Enlargement of the left supraclavicular lymph nodes, in association with carcinoma of the stomach.

Summary

ICE
▼
Inspect from the end of the bed
▼
Palpate the submental nodes
▼
Palpate the submandibular nodes
▼
Palpate the parotid nodes
▼
Palpate the pre-auricular node
▼
Palpate the posterior auricular nodes
▼
Palpate the occipital nodes
▼
Palpate the anterior border of the sternomastoid muscle
▼
Palpate the scalene node
▼
Palpate the supraclavicular fossa
▼
Palpate the posterior border of the sternomastoid
▼
Palpate the posterior triangle of the neck
▼
Examine other groups of lymph nodes (if appropriate)
▼
Examine the liver and spleen (if appropriate)
▼
Thank the patient
▼
Turn and face the examiner

Often patients suffer from the 'leper complex' and are very conscious of skin lesions. Therefore, it is important not to be reticent when examining skin lesions.

Wear gloves if appropriate, but remember that most skin lesions are not infective, and therefore not contagious.

ICE

- Introduce yourself.
- Consent the patient for the examination.
- Expose the necessary parts of the body and position the patient. This will obviously depend on the part of the body to be examined. Give the patient a hospital gown to wear if appropriate. If it facilitates your examination, ask the patient to wash off any make-up or to remove a wig.

Examination

Inspection

From the end of the bed

- Look around the bed for clues, eg creams, dressings, sunglasses, diabetic diets.
- Scan the patient from head to toe, and note:
  - Does the patient look well or unwell?
  - Does the patient have any obvious conditions, eg systemic sclerosis, dermatomyositis?
  - What is the patient's colour, eg pale, cyanosed, jaundiced, plethoric, slate-grey?

Skin lesions

Ensure that the skin to be examined is well illuminated (use a lamp if necessary).

Begin by looking at the part of the body presented by the patient, and note the features summarised in the box overleaf.

Features of skin lesions

• Primary lesion

• Secondary lesion

• Geometric shape, eg oval, circular, irregular

• Surface contour (see diagram opposite)

• Texture, eg rough, smooth, hard, soft

• Distribution, eg flexor, extensor surfaces

• Configuration of lesions

• Temperature, eg normal, hot

• Smell, eg odourless, foul-smelling

Primary lesion

The lesion should be described in dermatological terms. The following words are commonly used: macule; papule; nodule; plaque; vesicle; bulla; pustule; weal; purpura; ecchymosis; telangiectasia; cyst; comedo; burrow.

Secondary lesion

If present, the following should be described: crusting; scaling; excoriation; fissure; atrophy; striae; ulceration; lichenification; scarring.

If ulceration is present the following features should be noted or examined:

• Site

• Size

• Shape

• Edge (eg sharp, rolled)

• Wall (eg in-sloping, punched-out)

• Floor (eg granulation tissue)

• Base (eg mobile, sitting on bone)

• Details about the surrounding skin – both local and distant

• Regional lymph nodes (see cervical lymph nodes examination)

• Peripheral pulses near the lesion (see cardiovascular examination).

Surface contour

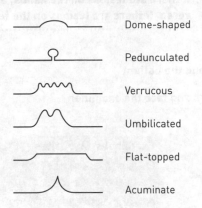

Dome-shaped

Pedunculated

Verrucous

Umbilicated

Flat-topped

Terms used to describe the
surface contour of a lesion

Acuminate

Configuration of lesions

Lesions are often found in certain configurations, as shown in the diagram.

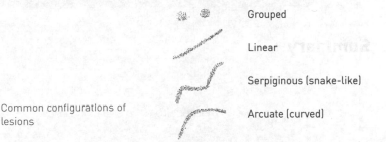

Grouped

Linear

Serpiginous (snake-like)

Common configurations of
lesions

Arcuate (curved)

Alternatively, the lesions may be scattered all over the body, in no particular
configuration.

**A simple diagram or photograph of the lesion is often useful for
recording details of the lesion, and monitoring how it may change over
time or in response to treatment.**

General skin examination

Ask about any other skin lesions present, and examine these. It may be
appropriate to look in the mouth for other signs of cutaneous disease, eg
Wickham's striae of lichen planus or white plaques of systemic candidiasis.

> **If there are lesions on the hands, always examine the feet, and vice versa. If there are lesions on the feet, always examine the groin.**

Thank the patient

Turn and face the examiner

Examiners' favourites

Q Name five skin diseases that may be associated with an underlying malignancy.

A Acanthosis nigricans, dermatomyositis, ichthyosis, migratory thrombophebitis, tylosis.

Q Name some risk factors for malignant melanoma.

A Celtic ancestry, sunburn, frequent sunbathing, multiple naevi, a history of skin neoplasia.

Summary

ICE
▼
Inspect from the end of the bed
▼
Examine any skin lesions
▼
Examine the skin generally
▼
Thank the patient
▼
Turn and face the examiner

Decide whether you want to examine the thyroid status of the patient or simply the thyroid gland itself. For the former, since thyroid dysfunction can be manifest in many body systems, it is necessary to examine more than just the gland.

ICE

- Introduce yourself.
- Consent the patient for the examination.
- Expose the necessary parts of the body and position the patient. Roll up the patient's sleeves, and loosen the collar to expose the neck. The patient should sit opposite the examiner on a chair if possible.

Examination

Inspection

From the end of the bed

- Look around the bed for clues of other disease.
- Scan the patient from head to toe, and note:
  - Does the patient look well or unwell?
  - Does the patient have any obvious conditions, eg Grave's disease?
  - Does the patient have any clues to thyroid disease that are immediately apparent, eg inappropriate dress for the temperature, irritability?
  - What is their weight?
  - Are they making any abnormal noises, eg stridor?

Hands

Take the patient's hands in yours and look for:

- onycholysis (nail lifting off the nail bed)
- palmar erythema
- excessive warmth or coldness
- sweatiness
- signs of carpal tunnel syndrome
- thyroid acropachy.

Test for tremor

Place a sheet of paper on top of the patient's outstretched hands. (This makes any tremor more obvious.)

Face

Look for:

- 'peaches and cream' complexion
- hair/eyebrow changes
- voice and tongue changes

Examine the radial pulse

Note the rate and rhythm.

Measure blood pressure (see cardiovascular examination for details)

Test for proximal myopathy in the arms

Press down on the patient's arms, which should be positioned in the same way as when you are testing the power of shoulder abductors (see peripheral nervous system examination).

Examine the eyes

- Inspect for:
  - exophthalmos (protrusion of the eye)
  - periorbital oedema.

Ⓥ **Inspect the eyes from above and from the sides.**

- Test eye movements (see eye examination).
- Watch for lid lag and lid retraction.

Inspect the neck

Inspect with the patient at rest, from the front and side, with the tongue in the mouth, protruded, and during swallowing. A thyroglossal cyst will move superiorly upon tongue protrusion.

Palpate the neck

Ⓥ **Ask the patient if their neck is sore before examining.**

- Stand behind the patient and palpate the whole thyroid gland.
- With one hand, stabilise one lateral lobe, and palpate the other lobe with the other hand.
- Repeat to examine the other lateral lobe.
- Finally, palpate both lobes simultaneously and ask the patient to swallow.

Check for cervical lymphadenopathy (see cervical lymph nodes examination).

Percuss the neck

Start at the suprasternal notch and work inferiorly. A large thyroid may extend retrosternally (this will be detected as dullness to percussion).

Auscultate the thyroid gland

• Listen over both lobes with the diaphragm of the stethoscope for bruits.

Ask the patient to breath-hold while you auscultate.

Test for proximal myopathy in the legs

Ask the patient to rise from a seated position, without using their hands.

Test the knee jerk reflexes (see peripheral nervous system)

Test for pretibial myxoedema

Press for up to 1 minute on the anterior aspect of the shin, and look for dimpling.

Thank the patient

Turn and face the examiner

Examiners' favourites

Q What signs of hypothyroidism might you detect on clinical examination?

A Overweight; peaches and cream complexion; cold hands; bradycardia; systolic hypertension; proximal myopathy; goitre; slow-relaxing (hung-up) reflexes.

Q What are the three signs unique to Graves' disease?

A Diffuse thyroid acropachy, ophthalmoplegia and pretibial myxoedema.

Summary

ICE
▼
Inspect from the end of the bed
▼
Inspect the hands
▼
Inspect the face
▼
Assess the radial pulse
▼
Measure the blood pressure
▼
Test for proximal myopathy in the arms
▼
Inspect the eyes
▼
Assess eye movements
▼
Inspect the neck
▼
Palpate the neck
▼
Percuss the neck
▼
Auscultate the thyroid gland
▼
Test for proximal myopathy in the legs
▼
Test the knee jerk reflexes
▼
Test for pretibial myxoedema
▼
Thank the patient
▼
Turn and face the examiner

It is important when carrying out this examination, to remember that this area is sensitive, and to appreciate that men may feel embarrassed and be afraid of getting hurt. Always carry out this examination very gently, and with concern for the patient's dignity.

ICE

- Introduce yourself.
- Consent the patient for the examination.
- Expose the necessary parts of the body and position the patient. The patient should be fully exposed from nipples to knees. Use a blanket to preserve dignity when you are not directly involved in examining. The patient should be lying flat on the bed, with the scrotum drawn forward to lie on the thighs.

Examination

Inspection
From the end of the bed

- Scan the patient from head to toe, and note:
  - Does the patient look well or unwell?
  - Does the patient have any obvious conditions, eg massive scrotal lump?

Scrotum

Inspect from all sides, and note the pubic hair distribution.

Palpation
Scrotum

Each side of the scrotum should be examined independently. Feel for lumps in the scrotal skin.

Spermatic cord

The spermatic cord should be palpated between finger and thumb, and its course followed from internal inguinal ring to testis.

Testes and epididymis

The testis and epididymis should be fully palpated. If measuring beads are available, the testicular size should be measured.

It is important to watch the patient's face during this part of the examination to ensure that you are not causing him any pain.

Inguinal regions

Palpate for lymphadenopathy.

Transillumination of a scrotal mass (only if a mass is palpated)

Shine a bright torch light at the back of the mass and note whether or not the light is transmitted. The torch should be shone through a tube held up against the mass, as shown in the diagram below.

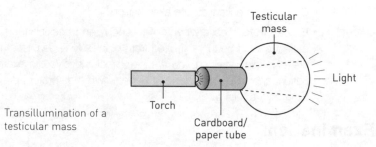

Testicular mass

Light

Transillumination of a testicular mass

Torch

Cardboard/ paper tube

Thank the patient

Cover the patient

Turn and face the examiner

Examiner's favourites

Q How might you differentiate between the various types of scrotal masses on examination?

A On finding a swelling, decide whether the swelling is on the scrotum or in the scrotum. If a mass is palpated in the scrotum, the key question to ask yourself is 'Can I get above it?' If it is not possible to feel the upper border of the mass, it is likely to be an inguinal hernia.

If you are able to palpate the upper border of the mass, you must then decide whether the mass is cystic or solid, and if it is separate from the testis or whether it lies within the testis. It is also possible that the testis may not be palpable because of the mass.

The final step should be to transilluminate the mass.

Noting the patient's age and taking a history are also important parts of deciding the cause of testicular pathology.

Q Which tumour markers are particularly relevant to testicular neoplasia?

A α-fetoprotein and β-human chorionic gonadotrophin.

Summary

ICE

▼

Inspect from the end of the bed

▼

Inspect the scrotum

▼

Palpate the scrotum

▼

Palpate the spermatic cords

▼

Palpate the testes and epididymis

▼

Palpate the inguinal regions

▼

Transilluminate any testicular masses

▼

Thank the patient

▼

Cover the patient

▼

Turn and face the examiner

Due to the intimate nature of this examination, it is imperative that it is carried out in as dignified a manner as possible.

Ⓥ **A female chaperone should always be present for this examination.**

Ⓥ **Always wear gloves.**

ICE

- **I**ntroduce yourself.
- **C**onsent the patient for the examination. It may be appropriate when obtaining consent to refer to the vagina as the 'front passage', since some patients may not be familiar with anatomical terminology.
- **E**xpose the necessary parts of the body and position the patient. Ask the patient to change into a hospital gown and to lie on the bed face up, bringing their feet up to their bottom, and letting the knees fall to the sides. Ensure that the area to be examined is adequately illuminated, using a lamp if necessary.

Examination

Inspection

From the end of the bed

Scan the patient from head to toe, and note:

- Does the patient look well or unwell?
- Does the patient have any obvious conditions, eg prolapsed uterus.

Genitalia

Note the following:

- Pubic hair
- Labia
- Clitoris
- Urethra
- Perianal area.

Pay particular attention to any swellings, discharge or bleeding.

Palpation

Ⓥ **Ask if there is any pain before beginning palpation, and watch the patient's face throughout the examination.**

- Part the labia majora using the index and middle fingers of your left hand in a 'scissor-like' motion. Ask the patient to cough, and look for any discharge or abnormalities of the vagina walls.
- Gently palpate Bartholin's glands (situated at the 5 and 7 o'clock positions of the labia). Normally, these cannot be palpated. Note any tenderness or swelling.
- If appropriate, gently 'milk' the urethra, and note the presence of any discharge.

Examination with a bivalve speculum

- Inform the patient that you are going to pass a small device into the front passage in order to look at the womb.
- Lubricate the speculum with some lubricating jelly. Inform the patient that you are about to insert the speculum.
- Pass the speculum slowly, with gentle pressure exerted backwards and downwards. Rotate the speculum as you insert in order to follow the contour of the vagina. The device should be inserted in a vertical plane, and rotated to lie in a horizontal plane.
- When it is in position, open the speculum out, and inspect the cervix. Look at the shape and size of the cervix, and note any abnormalities, such as erosions, polyps or discharge.
- Tell the patient that you are going to remove the speculum, before doing so slowly and gently.

Bimanual examination

- Inform the patient that you are going to insert two fingers into the front passage in order to feel the womb.
- Lubricate the index and middle fingers of your gloved right hand. Pass the fingers in gently. Rotate the fingers as you insert in order to follow the contour of the vagina. The fingers should be inserted in a vertical plane, and rotated to lie in a horizontal plane.
- Feel the cervix with the tips of your fingers.
- Using your left hand, palpate the abdomen starting near the xiphisternum, and work downwards. Try to feel the uterus between your two hands. Assess its size, shape, motility and tenderness. It may be possible to palpate the ovaries also, and any tenderness or other abnormalities should be noted.
- Tell the patient that you are going to remove your fingers, before doing so slowly and gently.
- Clean any lubricating jelly from the patient with a tissue.

Thank the patient

Cover the patient

Turn and face the examiner

> **Examiners' favourites**
>
> **Q** What does the current UK cervical screening programme entail?
>
> **A** All women aged between 25 and 64 are eligible for cervical screening every 3 to 5 years. A cervical smear or liquid-based cytology is used to examine cervical cells for malignant or pre-malignant changes. The frequency of cervical screening depends on a patient's age and on whether or not any abnormalities have been detected in the past.
>
> **Q** Name three risk factors for cervical cancer.
>
> **A** Exposure to human papillomavirus (especially type 16), young age at first coitus, multiple sexual partners.

Summary

ICE

▼

Inspect from the end of the bed

▼

Inspect the genitalia

▼

Palpate Bartholin's glands

▼

'Milk' the urethra if appropriate

▼

Perform a bivalve speculum examination

▼

Perform a bimanual examination

▼

Thank the patient

▼

Cover the patient

▼

Turn and face the examiner

A rectal examination may be carried out as part of a complete alimentary system examination, or in isolation.

> **Because of the intimate nature of this examination, it is imperative that the examination is carried out in as dignified a manner as possible.**

> **A chaperone should always be present for this examination.**

> **Always wear gloves.**

ICE

- Introduce yourself.
- Consent the patient for the examination. It is recommended that the rectum is referred to as 'the back passage' when obtaining consent, since some patients may not be familiar with anatomical terminology. Explain that the procedure may be uncomfortable, but it should not be painful.
- Expose the necessary part of the body and position the patient: Ask the patient to change into a hospital gown and to lie on the bed on the left side (left lateral position). They should then bring the knees up as close to the chest as possible, trying to get into the position where the buttocks are as close to the edge of the couch as possible. Ensure that the area to be examined is adequately illuminated, using a lamp if necessary.

Examination

Inspection

From the end of the bed

Scan the patient from head to toe, and note:

- Does the patient look well or unwell?
- Does the patient have any obvious conditions, eg prolapsed rectum?

Perianal area

Expose the perianal area by lifting up the right buttock. Look for:

- fissures
- haemorrhoids
- skin tags or rashes

- warts
- fistulae.

Ask the patient to 'strain down', and note any rectal prolapse.

Palpation

- Lubricate the index finger of your gloved right hand using lubricating jelly.
- Touch the perianal area gently, and test light touch sensation on the perineum and perianal skin.
- Tell the patient that you are going to insert your finger. Gently insert your index finger into the rectum, so that the palmar aspect of the finger is oriented towards the patient's back. Note the tone of the anal sphincter muscle as you insert your finger. Palpate the rectal wall with your finger. Watch the patient's face for any signs of pain during the examination.
- Gently and slowly, rotate your hand anticlockwise and palpate the rectal wall until the palmar aspect of your finger is facing the patient's front. Then, rotate your hand in a clockwise direction until the finger is back in the starting position. Continue to rotate the hand in a clockwise direction until the palmar aspect of the finger is again facing the patient's front. Withdraw the finger slightly, and ask the patient to strain down again. Palpate the lower rectum for any abnormalities.
- Tell the patient that you are now going to remove your finger, and do so slowly.

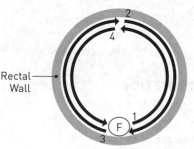

Rectal Wall

Path taken during palpation of the rectal wall.
F = finger starting point

At the end of the examination, all areas of the rectal wall should have been palpated.

> **Particular attention should be paid to the prostate gland in male patients. This is palpated through the anterior wall of the rectum.**

The glove should be inspected on withdrawal for the presence of blood, mucus, stools, or other abnormality. Clean any lubricating jelly from the patient with a tissue.

Thank the patient

Cover the patient

Turn and face the examiner

> **Examiners' favourites**
>
> **Q** How would you distinguish between a benign and a malignant prostatic tumour on examination?
>
> **A** Benign: smooth surface; sulcus felt. Malignant: irregular, craggy border; loss of medial sulcus.
>
> **Q** Which blood test would you order if you suspected prostate cancer?
>
> **A** Prostate specific antigen (PSA).

Summary

ICE
▼
Inspect from the end of the bed
▼
Inspect the perianal area
▼
Test perineal and perianal sensation
▼
Palpate the rectum
▼
Thank the patient
▼
Cover the patient
▼
Turn and face the examiner

For obvious reasons, the usual ICE approach is not applicable when testing the level of consciousness.

Consciousness is a state of awareness of one's self and the surrounding environment. In most medical consultations, the level of consciousness is not formally assessed. Patients are fully conscious if they can co-operate with history-taking and examination. However, the level of consciousness can alter, especially in the emergency setting, and such a change is often indicative of a serious pathological process.

The level of detail with which one assesses and records the level of consciousness depends on the medical setting. Three methods for assessing consciousness level are described below.

In order to elicit pain for the purposes of these assessments, use one of three recognised methods:

- Apply pressure over the sternum using the knuckles of your clenched hand;
- Using the thumb, apply pressure over the supraorbital ridge (the top of the eye socket); or
- Use the barrel of a pen to exert pressure on a nailbed.

Method 1

This is the simplest and most applicable to use on a general ward. Score the patient from 0 to 5 using the following scale:

- 5: fully conscious and alert
- 4: confused, but responding appropriately
- 3: obeying vocal commands
- 2: semi-purposeful movement to pain
- 1: reflex movement to pain (withdrawal)
- 0: unresponsive to pain.

Levels 3 and 4 may be referred to as 'clouding of consciousness'. Level 2 may be considered as 'stupor', whereas levels 1 and 0 represent a state of 'coma'.

Method 2

An extremely basic and rapid system – AVPU – is often used in emergency medicine:

- **A**lert
- responds to **V**oice
- responds to **P**ain
- **U**nconscious

Method 3

It may be necessary to perform a more detailed and formal assessment of a patient's conscious state, especially in emergency or intensive-care departments. This can be done by using the Glasgow Coma Scale (GCS). Three key areas are assessed: eye-opening, best motor response and best verbal response. The patient is given a score for each category, and the sum of these scores represents the patient's GCS score.

The minimum score is 3 and the maximum is 15.

Eye-opening

1 None

2 Open with pain

3 Open on verbal command

4 Open spontaneously

Best motor response

1 None

2 Abnormal extension with pain

3 Abnormal flexion with pain

4 Weak flexion withdrawal from pain

5 Localising pain

6 Obeying commands

Best verbal response

1 None

2 Incomprehensible speech

3 Inappropriate speech

4 Confused speech

5 Orientated

Examiners' favourites

Q What is the minimum score in the Glasgow Coma Scale?

A 3 out of 15

Q What is the first blood test that should be performed in a patient who is found unconcious

A Blood glucose (generally tested with a capillary blood glucose sampling kit).

The mental state examination is the psychiatric equivalent of a physical examination. When the presenting complaint is primarily one relating to mental health, a detailed formal assessment is undertaken. For the purposes of a general health assessment it is sufficient to use the Mini Mental State format as detailed below. This follows a standardised system, giving a score out of 30.

Many routinely examine the mental state when assessing the elderly patient.

> **Each * symbol below indicates what constitutes 1 point scored for a correct answer.**

ICE

- Introduce yourself.
- Consent the patient for the examination (eg 'I would like to ask you some questions to test your memory. Is that OK?').
- Exposure not needed. The patient should sit opposite you on a chair or bed.

Orientation

- Can you tell me today's date*, month* and year*?
- Which day of the week is it today*?
- Can you also tell me which season it is*?
- What city/town are we in*?
- What county* and country*?
- What building are we in* and on what floor*?

Anterograde (short-term) memory

- I would like you to remember three objects (orange, tobacco, airplane).
- Ask for the words to be repeated (registration) and score 1 for each correct word***.
- Repeat until all three are remembered, allowing up to six attempts. Record the number of trials needed.

Attention and calculation

- Serial 7s. Starting with the number 100, subtract 7 and repeat, ie 100, 93, 86... Stop at 65. Score 1 for each correct number*****.

- Alternatively, for those who have a dislike for numbers, ask them to spell the word 'WORLD' backwards. Score 1 for each letter*****.

> **Note that only one of the above tests should be carried out.**

Recall

- What are the three words I asked you to remember earlier (orange, tobacco, airplane)? Score 1 for each correct word remembered***.

Language

- Name these objects (show the patient two easily recognisable objects, eg watch, pen)**.
- Repeat the following phrase: 'no ifs, ands or buts'*.
- Read this sentence and do what it says. (Show card with 'CLOSE YOUR EYES' written on it). Score 1 if the patient closes their eyes*.
- Write a short, simple sentence (eg 'I went to the shops yesterday')*.
- Take this piece of paper in your left hand*, fold it in half* and put it on the floor*.
- Can you copy this drawing (both pentagons must have five sides and overlap)*?

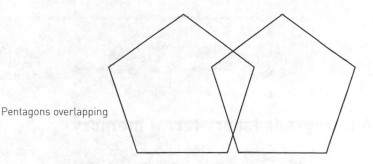

Pentagons overlapping

> **These six aspects of language test, respectively: naming, repeating, reading, writing, three-stage-command and visuospatial components.**

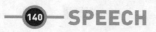

ICE

- **I**ntroduce yourself.
- **C**onsent the patient for the examination.
- **E**xposure not necessary here.

Assess the speech

Follow the flow diagram to assess the speech. See opposite for directions on how to test each stage.

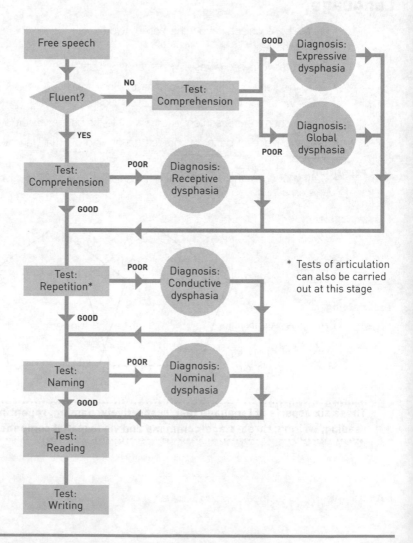

* Tests of articulation can also be carried out at this stage

Free speech

Try to get the patient talking. Ask them why they are in hospital, or to describe a typical day.

Comprehension

- Comprehending one-step commands that are spoken. Ask the patient to:
  - close the eyes
  - stick out the tongue.
- Comprehending complex commands that are spoken. Ask the patient to:
  - cover the right eye with the left hand
  - touch their left knee with the left hand.
- Comprehending language. Ask the patient:
  - whether he puts on a tie before a shirt or whether she puts on shoes before stockings
  - whether a car is a type of animal.
- Comprehending written commands:
  - write a command, eg 'close your eyes', on a piece of paper, and ask the patient to do as it states.

Test repetition

Make up a sentence, and ask the patient to repeat it to you.

Test articulation

Ask the patient to repeat some phrases after you, such as:

- British constitution
- baby hippopotamus.

Test naming

Ask the patient to name an object that you show, eg tie, pen, watch.

Test further by asking the patient to name the parts of an object, eg hands and strap of a watch.

Examiners' favourites

Q What is the anatomical location of the two main speech areas in the brain?

A Broca's area – posterior 3rd frontal gyrus on the dominant hemisphere.
Wernicke's area – posterior 1st temporal gyrus on the dominant hemisphere.

Q What abnormalities of speech might be present in a patient with cerebellar disease?

A Explosive, staccato speech which is usually loud.

ICE

- Introduce yourself.
- Consent the patient for the examination.
- Expose the necessary parts of the body and position the patient. Roll up any trouser legs to expose the ankles. Position the back of the bed at 45° to the horizontal.

Examination

Inspection

From the end of the bed

- Look around the bed for clues, eg fluid restriction signs, nutritional supplements, a urine collection bag.
- Scan the patient from head to toe, and note:
  - Does the patient look well or unwell?
  - Does the patient have any obvious conditions, eg Prader–Willi syndrome?
  - Does the patient have obviously swollen ankles?
  - What is the patient's colour, eg pale, cyanosed, jaundiced, ruddy complexion?

Face

In severe dehydration, the eyes may appear 'sunken'.

Ask the patient to open their mouth, then inspect the tongue and mucous membranes for moisture. Dehydration will cause these surfaces to appear dry.

Speak to the patient

Stimulating thirst is one of the body's usual responses to dehydration, so ask the patient if they are thirsty. One may also smell the fetor of dehydration.

Test capillary refill time

Raise the thumb to the level of the heart, and press hard on the pulp. Press for 5 seconds, and then release. Time how long it takes the pink colour to return to the patient's digit. Normally, this should be less than 2 seconds. A prolonged capillary refill time indicates poor blood supply to the peripheries.

Measure the pulse rate

Tachycardia (pulse > 100 beats per minute) may occur either if the patient is dehydrated or if they are fluid-overloaded.

Measure the blood pressure lying and standing

Hypotension (low blood pressure) is a common feature of dehydration. A postural drop in blood pressure would also be in keeping with dehydration.

Assess skin turgor

Using your thumb and index finger, gently pinch the patient's skin on the forearm. With normal hydration, the skin will promptly return to its original position. In dehydration, skin turgor is reduced, and the skin takes longer to return to its original state.

Assess the JVP

The height of the JVP is usually low in dehydration, but raised with fluid overload.

Auscultate the lungs

Pulmonary oedema occurs with severe fluid overload. This will commonly be manifest as fine inspiratory crepitations (crackles) in the bases of the lungs.

Test for pitting oedema

Ask the patient to sit forward. Press on the skin over the sacrum to test for sacral oedema. Test also for ankle oedema. Oedema often occurs with fluid overload in right heart failure. However, it is also associated with prolonged bed rest and low protein levels in the blood.

Thank the patient

Turn to the examiner

State that you would like to complete the examination by:

- inspecting the patient's fluid balance chart
- performing urinalysis – in normal circumstances, the urine is concentrated with dehydration, and dilute with fluid overload.

Examiners' favourites

Q How is total body water usually distributed in an adult?

A Two thirds is intracellular fluid. The remaining third is extracellular. Of this one quarter is in the plasma.

Q Name some common causes of bilateral pitting ankle oedema.

A Right heart failure, constrictive pericarditis, hypoalbuminaemia (eg. in liver cirrhosis, nephrotic syndrome, malabsorption or protein-loosing enteropathy).

Summary

ICE

▼

Inspect from the end of the bed

▼

Inspect the face

▼

Enquire about thirst

▼

Test capillary refill time

▼

Measure the pulse rate

▼

Measure the blood pressure lying and standing

▼

Assess skin turgor

▼

Assess the JVP

▼

Auscultate the lungs

▼

Test for pitting oedema

▼

Thank the patient

▼

Turn and face the examiner

SECTION 3
PRACTICAL PROCEDURES

Venous cannulation is an essential skill for any junior doctor. A significant percentage of hospitalised patients will require intravenous access for the administration of fluids and medications.

A venous cannula may be inserted into just about any vein, although, conventional insertion sites include the forearm and dorsum of the hand. There are a range of cannula sizes available. For routine purposes in an adult patient, a 20-gauge cannula will suffice. However, the size of the cannula influences the speed with which fluids can be administered. Therefore, in emergency situations the largest cannula available should be inserted if possible.

In a number of patients, peripheral cannulation may be unachievable – especially those with multiple previous admissions, intravenous drug abusers and those receiving regular cytotoxic medications. In these circumstances two main options are available: external jugular vein cannulation or central line insertion. Both should be undertaken only by experienced practitioners. The procedure for external jugular vein cannulation is included at the end of this section.

Indications for venous cannulation

For administration of:

- IV fluids
- IV medications
- blood products
- inotropic agents*
- parenteral feeds*

* Central access only

Patients with chronic renal failure may require the formation of a fistula in the future. In these patients, cannulae should only usually be inserted into the dorsum of the hand. Under no circumstances should a cannula be inserted into a fistula.

Equipment

- 5 ml of 0.9% saline (for a flush)
- Antiseptic wipes
- Cannulae
- Cotton-wool balls
- Dressing (to fix cannula in place)
- Gloves
- Tourniquet.

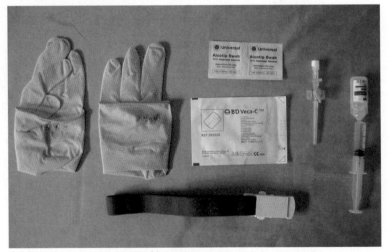

Equipment for forearm venous cannulation

ICE

- **I**ntroduce yourself.
- **C**onsent the patient for the procedure.
- **E**xpose the necessary parts of the body and position the patient. Roll up the patient's sleeve to well above the elbow. For external jugular vein cannulation, tilt the bed to 10–15° head-down.

Procedures

Forearm vein cannulation

- Wash your hands.
- Apply a tourniquet around the arm, above the elbow. Alternatively, a blood

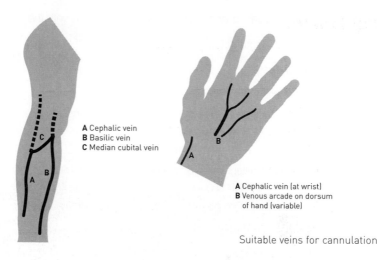

A Cephalic vein
B Basilic vein
C Median cubital vein

A Cephalic vein (at wrist)
B Venous arcade on dorsum
of hand (variable)

Suitable veins for cannulation

pressure cuff may be used. The cuff should be inflated to exert a pressure somewhere between the diastolic and systolic blood pressure. This will allow the veins to distend by engorgement.

- Assess the forearm for suitably engorged veins for cannulation.
- The best veins to cannulate are those that you can both see and feel.
- Gloves should be worn for venepuncture; however, you may wish to feel the vein initially without gloves, especially with the more difficult cannulations.
- Clean the chosen area for cannulation with an antiseptic wipe. A site just proximal to the union of two veins is often a secure spot. Inform the patient of a 'small scratch'. If the patient is likely to move the arm, request assistance from the nursing staff to fix the arm.

Union point of veins

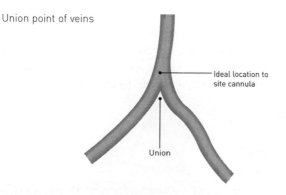

Ideal location to
site cannula

Union

- Make a clean, assertive pass at a shallow angle with the cannula.
- When the cannula enters the vein, there will be a flashback of blood.
- At this point, advance the cannula while simultaneously withdrawing the needle.
- When it is fully inserted, release the tourniquet.
- Apply pressure at the proximal end of the cannula to prevent leakage of blood and apply the cap to its distal end.
- Fix the cannula in place with a dressing.
- Check the patency of the cannula by flushing it will 5 ml of 0.9% saline. A properly inserted cannula will not leak, and flushing it will not cause any pain.
- Dispose of all sharps carefully in a suitable container.
- Wash your hands.

External jugular vein cannulation

This may be considered in emergency scenarios where venous access is essential, but no peripheral access is possible and circumstances do not allow for immediate central line placement. Successful placement will depend on the availability of a suitable vein.

- To ensure the best of chance of observing a candidate vein, the patient should be tilted to 10–15° head-down to allow the veins to engorge. The external jugular vein crosses the sternomastoid muscle in the neck.
- The neck should be prepared aseptically by cleaning with iodine or chlorhexidine.

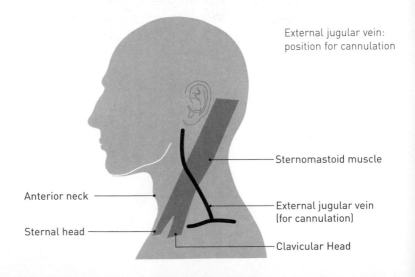

External jugular vein: position for cannulation

Sternomastoid muscle

Anterior neck

External jugular vein (for cannulation)

Sternal head

Clavicular Head

- A subcutaneous bleb of 1–2 ml of 1% lidocaine should be infiltrated around the chosen spot for insertion.
- Choose the largest cannula available (ideally a 16- or 14-gauge), and attach a 5ml syringe to the back portion, following removal of the cap.
- Ask the patient to rotate the head away from the chosen side of the neck.
- Position oneself at the head of the bed.
- Cannulate as described for a peripheral location but you should aspirate on the attached 5ml syringe at the point of insertion.
- Correct placement will be confirmed by the aspiration of venous blood.
- Advance the cannula smoothly as for peripheral insertion.
- Fix the cannula in place with a dressing.
- Flush the line with 0.9% saline to maintain its patency.
- Dispose of all sharps carefully in a suitable container.
- Wash your hands.

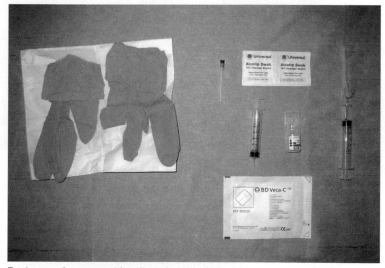

Equipment for external jugular vein cannulation

Arterial blood gas sampling is a commonly requested test in an acutely unwell hospital patient. It is invasive and may be unpleasant for the patient; however, it is often vital in dictating management.

Conventional blood gas analysis provides the pH, PaO_2, $PaCO_2$, bicarbonate and base excess. In some machines, and when clinically indicated, indices such as lactate and methaemoglobin may be measured.

Outside an intensive-care environment, arterial blood gas sampling requires an arterial 'stab' from the radial artery. In difficult cases or acute emergencies, the femoral artery or, more rarely, the brachial artery may be used. Both radial and femoral approaches are described here.

Equipment

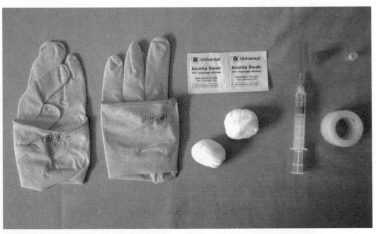

Equipment for arterial blood gas sampling

- 2ml heparinised syringe
- Antiseptic wipe
- Cotton-wool balls
- Cup full of ice (if sample not being analysed instantly)
- Gloves
- Needle
- Syringe bung
- Tape.

An arterial blood gas sampling kit is commonly available, containing a heparinised syringe, needle and bung.

ICE

- Introduce yourself.
- Consent the patient for the procedure. It is a good idea to inform the unsuspecting patient that this is a little different from venepuncture with which they may be familiar, usually being considerably more uncomfortable.
- Expose the necessary part of the body and position the patient. To obtain a radial artery sample, roll up the patient's sleeve. Ensure the patient's forearm is well supported. The placement of a pillow or a 500ml bag of fluid may help to support the wrist, maintaining it at a neutral or slightly extended position. For a femoral artery sample, the groin should be adequately exposed. The patient must be lying supine with the hip extended.

Procedures

Radial artery sample

- Wash your hands.
- Locate the chosen artery for sampling by feeling for a radial pulse at the wrist.
- Don a pair of gloves and clean the chosen site with an antiseptic wipe.
- In difficult cases you may wish at this stage to locate the pulse again and keep a single finger adjacent to the chosen site to aid direction for puncture. If the skin over this area is slack or you suspect the patient may move the forearm, ask for assistance to fix the forearm.
- In some circumstances it may be appropriate to first inject a small volume of lidocaine subcutaneously at the chosen site.

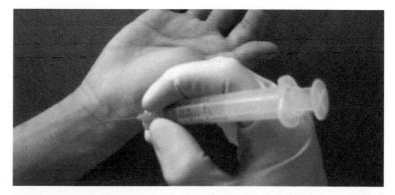

Radial artery sampling

- Make a confident, firm pass of the needle into the artery at approximately 45° to the skin surface. Confirmation of a successful arterial puncture will be seen as blood flashes back into the needle and syringe.

- If difficulties are encountered, withdraw the needle, so that the tip is just under the skin. Then re-insert with an appropriate change of angle.

- When a sufficient sample volume has been obtained (1–2 ml), withdraw the needle and apply firm pressure to the puncture site for at least 1 minute.

- Fix a cotton-wool ball tightly to the site using tape.

- Dispose of all sharps carefully in a suitable container.

- Wash your hands.

Take care initially to locate the pulse most amenable to puncture.

Ensure that pressure is applied for at least 1 minute and a tightly applied dressing is added afterwards to prevent the formation of a haematoma.

Femoral artery sample

When you are unable to obtain an arterial blood gas from elsewhere (for example during a cardiac arrest with no cardiac output), a sample may be taken from the large femoral artery.

This artery is accessible halfway between the anterior superior iliac spine and the pubic symphysis – the mid-inguinal point. This approximately equates to the upper lateral border of the pubic hair in most adults. The artery lies between the femoral nerve and femoral vein in the femoral triangle. It should be strongly palpable. A long needle (21-gauge) is usually required, particularly in patients with a large body habitus.

The procedure is carried out in a similar fashion to radial artery sampling. The pressure with which the blood enters the syringe will confirm arterial rather than venous blood. Apply pressure for at least 5 minutes post-procedure to prevent haematoma formation.

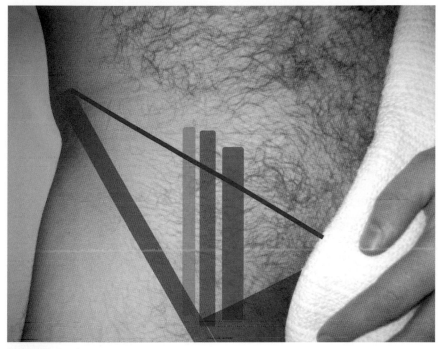

Femoral triangle

Placement of a nasogastric (NG) tube is a common procedure in both medical and surgical inpatients. There are a number of indications for its placement, including the removal of secretions and the facilitation of enteral nutrition. The co-operation of the patient is essential for quick, successful placement; however, in many circumstances, this may be lacking.

Equipment

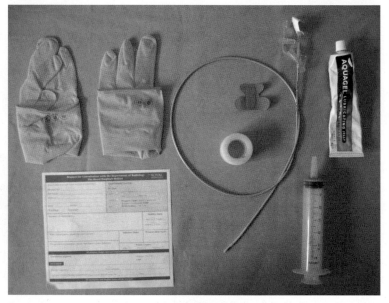

Equipment for placement of nasogastric tube

- 50ml syringe
- Aqueous gel
- Cup of water (optional)
- Chest X-ray request form
- Gloves
- Litmus paper
- NG tube (feeding or wide-bore)
- Plaster/tape.

ICE

- **I**ntroduce yourself.
- **C**onsent the patient for the procedure.
- **E**xpose the necessary part of the body and position the patient. Sit the patient forward with the neck slightly flexed.

Procedure

- Check the patency of the nasal meati. Choose the most suitable side for the passage of the tube.
- Estimate the length of tube required for passage into the stomach by measuring the distance from the mouth to the epigastrium.
- Wash your hands and put on a pair of gloves.
- Apply an ample amount of gel around the meatus and the first 4cm of the NG tube.
- Insert the tube into the nasal meatus and, using gentle pressure, advance the tube downwards and backwards towards the nasopharynx.
- If appropriate, ask the patient to take a sip of water and swallow. Alternatively, if the patient is not permitted to drink, ask them to make a swallowing action. These measures assist in the passage of the tube over the tongue.
- Continue to feed the tube in until the required length has been inserted.
- Secure the tube in place by applying tape (or the specially shaped plaster often supplied with NG tube kits) to fix it at the nasal meatus. Fix any excess tubing to the side of the patient's face.
- Confirm the correct position of the tube. Aspirate with a 50ml syringe from the port of the tube. Test the pH of the aspirate with litmus paper. An acidic aspirate provides evidence that the tube is in the stomach. Note if the patient is taking acid suppressant drugs.
- If the NG tube is being used for feeding or if there is any doubt as to the tube's position, a chest X-ray should be requested to confirm the tube's location. Do not allow the tube to be used until this has been reviewed by a trained member of staff.
- Wash your hands.

Ensure an ample amount of gel is applied to both the nasal meatus and the initial 4 cm of the NG tube to ensure smooth passage.

Invariably, the most difficult part is passing the tube over the back of the tongue and into the upper pharynx.

In the unco-operative patient, it is not uncommon for the tube to curl up within the mouth. Check for this during the procedure.

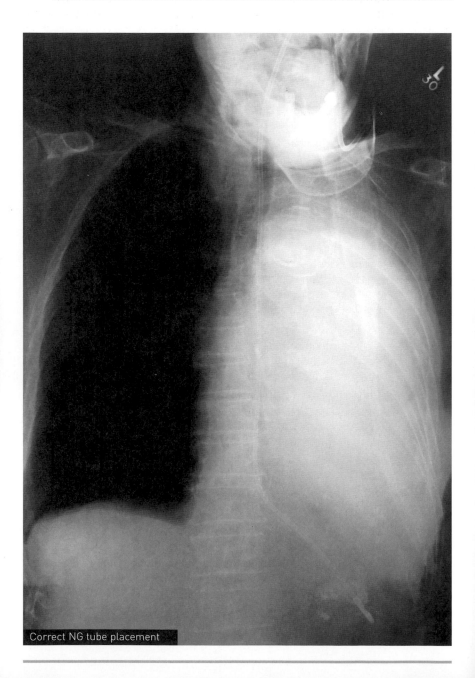

Correct NG tube placement

While female catheterisation is undertaken almost exclusively by nursing staff, male urinary catheterisation remains largely in the domain of the doctor. This procedure must be justifiable before it is undertaken, given the potential, albeit small, risk of complications. Documentation of the procedure within the medical notes, particularly any unexpected or difficult elements, is essential.

Aseptic technique is vital to prevent the introduction of infection, with particular care required for recatheterisation. A single dose of prophylactic antibiotics is indicated in these circumstances (usually in the form of intravenous gentamicin).

Equipment

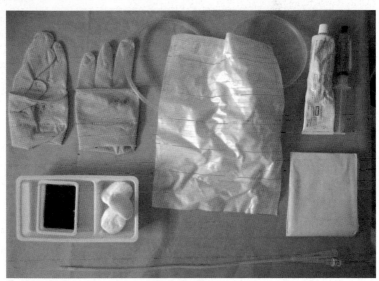

Equipment for male urinary catheterisation

- 10ml of sterile water in a syringe (for balloon inflation)
- Dressing pack
- Antiseptic fluid (usually chlorhexidine)
- Cotton-wool balls
- Sterile drape
- Sterile gloves
- Tube of lidocaine gel (10 ml)
- Urinary catheter (14-gauge initially in adult male)
- Urine collection bag or hourly urometer.

ICE

- **I**ntroduce yourself.
- **C**onsent the patient for the procedure.
- **E**xpose the necessary part and position the patient: the patient should lie supine, and should be exposed from umbilicus to knee.

Procedure

- Wash your hands and put on sterile gloves.
- Request for each piece of the equipment (listed above) to be handed to you in turn in an aseptic manner.
- Take the sterile drape and make a hole just big enough to pass the penis through. Place this appropriately over the patient.
- Retract the foreskin.
- Using cotton-wool balls soaked in antiseptic fluid, liberally clean the glans penis and beneath the foreskin. You may need to remove any smegma to make a clean field. Hold the penis with one hand to facilitate this process if necessary. Ideally, the penis should be held with a piece of sterile gauze to avoid contamination of your sterile glove.
- Hold the penis with one hand, and insert the tip of the lidocaine gel tube into the urethral meatus. Gently insert the gel, encouraging it to pass down the urethra. The gel offers both anaesthesia and lubrication to insert the catheter.
- Allow around 1 minute for the gel to take effect. Squeeze the urethra at the base of the glans to prevent the gel from escaping, and then remove the gel tube.

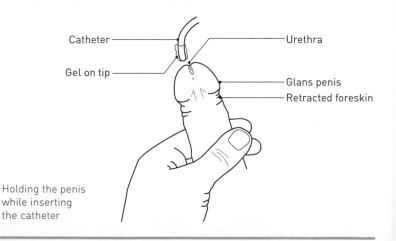

Catheter ———— ——— Urethra

Gel on tip ————

———— Glans penis
———— Retracted foreskin

Holding the penis
while inserting
the catheter

- Continue to hold the penis with one hand, and use your other hand to pass the catheter into the penis. Catheters usually pass most easily when the penis is held vertically (ie tip pointing towards the ceiling).
- Continue inserting until either urine flows back through the catheter tubing or a reasonable length of catheter has been passed (this may vary between patients). If there is any difficulty with the passage of the catheter, do not persist. There may be a particular problem at the level of the prostatic urethra in older patients.
- Attach the urine collection bag to the catheter.
- Inflate the balloon with 10 ml of water, watching the patient's face throughout for pain, which indicates incorrect placement of the balloon. If pain is present, deflate the balloon, remove the catheter and start again.
- Replace the foreskin.
- Note the residual volume of urine. Do not allow a distended bladder to decompress too quickly as this may lead to haemorrhage from vessels within the bladder muscle.
- Wash your hands.
- Document the procedure in the medical notes (as outlined below).

Always replace the foreskin post-procedure to prevent phimosis.

Documentation of catheterisation

An accurate medical note is essential. For example:

12/3/2004, 15.00 hours, P. Smyth (PRHO)

Urinary catheterisation
- Indication: congestive cardiac failure on diuretic therapy, for accurate output measurement
- Aseptic technique
- 14-gauge silastic catheter passed freely
- 10ml of water into balloon
- Foreskin replaced
- Residual volume: 250ml.

Lumbar puncture can be performed in an acute setting or electively for chronic neurological symptoms. Once the decision for this procedure to be undertaken has been made, there must be clinical plus/minus radiological confidence that the intracranial pressure is not raised. In the presence of a raised intracranial pressure, a lumbar puncture could be potentially fatal. Lumbar puncture requires a co-operative patient.

A lumbar puncture should not be performed if there is any suspicion of raised intracranial pressure.

Indications for lumbar puncture

- Diagnosis of a neurological infection (meningitis and encephalitis)
- Supportive diagnosis of demyelinating disease (multiple sclerosis)
- Clinically suspected subarachnoid haemorrhage, despite normal brain imaging (to look for xanthochromia)
- Diagnosis of rarer neurological disease (eg Lyme disease, neurosarcoidosis, neuromalignancy)

Equipment

- 5ml syringe
- 5 ml of 1% lidocaine
- Antiseptic fluid (chlorhexidine and iodine)
- Dressing pack

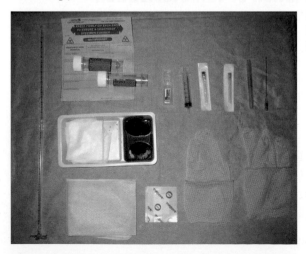

Equipment for lumbar puncture

- Manometer
- Orange (25-gauge) and green (21-gauge) needles
- Simple dressing
- Spinal needle (20-gauge most commonly used)*
- Sterile bottles (as many as required for samples)
- Sterile gloves.

* Dependent to an extent on patient's body habitus.

ICE

- **I**ntroduce yourself.
- **C**onsent the patient for the procedure. Inform the patient of the potential complications of the procedure, the most common being a headache and mild back discomfort. Formal written consent is required.
- **E**xpose the necessary part of the body and position the patient. The lumbar part of the back needs to be exposed, which will require both the shirt and trousers to be loosened and moved away from the field of work. Alternatively, ask the patient to remove these items as deemed appropriate. Position the patient in the left lateral position, ie lying on the left-hand side. Ask the patient to raise the knees towards the chin ('like a fetus in a mother's tummy'). The back should be kept as straight as possible and be as close to the edge of the bed as is safely feasible. In some circumstances you may need to move the patient into the correct position if they are unable to co-operate. Adjust the bed to a comfortable height for you to perform the procedure while seated.

Procedure

- With the patient positioned, try to avoid further repositioning once you have started to palpate the intervertebral space.

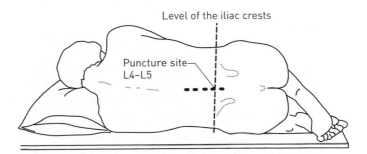

Left lateral position for lumbar puncture with line from iliac crests through L4

- Palpate for the right iliac crest – this may be more difficult in overweight patients. The plane of the iliac crests is through the level of L4.

The spinal cord ends at L2 in the adult.

- Palpate for the intervertebral space between either L3/4 or L4/5. This may be harder to feel in those with spinal abnormalities, such as degenerative disc disease.
- Mark the preferred spot with an indentation of the finger nail.
- Wash your hands and put on a pair of sterile gloves.
- Clean the area around the chosen spot with iodine and chlorhexidine.
- Infiltrate the skin with a small subcutaneous bleb (0.5–1 ml) of lidocaine at the chosen spot with the 25-gauge needle. Change the needle to the 21-gauge needle and, passing through the bleb in the skin in a plane towards the umbilicus, infiltrate further in the tract that the spinal needle will follow. This allows you to gain a feel for the space (softer but firm, compared with the bony vertebrae).
- Prepare the spinal needle. Insert the spinal needle, bevel up, in a plane towards the umbilicus. The depth to which the needle will need to be passed will depend on the patient's habitus.
- It may be difficult initially to pass the spinal needle through the skin. Firm pressure may be required. There will be a 'pop' or a 'giving way' as the needle passes through the dura and into the subarachnoid space.
- Withdraw the stylette. The cerebrospinal fluid (CSF) should then flow freely back through the needle. If not, reposition as appropriate. This may require withdrawing the needle to just before (but not out of) the skin before you can re-angle the needle for a further pass.
- Place the manometer onto the spinal needle and measure the CSF pressure. Normal opening pressure should be 10–20 cmH$_2$O. The three-way tap can then be manipulated to collect the CSF within the manometer into the tubes.
- Collect 10–15 drops into each sterile bottle. Label each bottle in the order that they were used.
- Withdraw the spinal needle and place a simple dressing over the wound.
- Advise the patient to remain supine for at least an hour in an attempt to minimise post-lumbar puncture headache.
- Send the CSF sample for appropriate analysis (see box).
- Document the procedure in the medical notes, as detailed below.
- Wash your hands.

CSF analysis

Routine analyses

- Microbiology (white cell count, including differential, erythrocytes, organisms, culture and sensitivity)

- Total protein

- Glucose*

* A concurrent plasma glucose is essential to calculate the CSF:plasma glucose ratio. This is usually greater than two-thirds.

Additional analyses

- Oligoclonal bands (not unique to multiple sclerosis, but present in > 95%)

- Xanthochromia in suspected subarachnoid haemorrhage

- Neuropathology for cells

- Herpes simplex/zoster PCR serology

- Protein 14-3-3 (variant Creutzfeldt–Jacob disease)

- *Borrelia burgdorferi* serology (Lyme disease)

Correct positioning is essential for a straightforward lumbar puncture. It maximises the size of the intervertebral space.

Documentation of lumbar puncture

21/5/2004, 16.00 hours, I. Yunos (Medical SHO)

Diagnostic lumbar puncture

- Indication: clinical suspicion of bacterial meningitis

- Consent obtained

- Aseptic technique

- 3 ml of 1% lidocaine infiltrated subcutaneously

- 1st pass L3–4 intervertebral space

- Opening pressure 18 cm H_2O

- CSF: turbid appearance

- CSF sent for: microbiology, total protein, glucose

- Associated serum sample sent for total protein and glucose.

A pleural effusion is an abnormal collection of fluid within the pleural cavity for which there are many causes. As part of the assessment of patients with this problem, analysis of the pleural fluid may be of benefit. Large pleural effusions may cause shortness of breath and therefore therapeutic aspiration can be undertaken for symptomatic benefit. Be particularly careful in those with limited respiratory reserve because of the risk of pneumothorax.

Equipment

- Dressing pack
- Antiseptic fluid (usually chlorhexidine) and iodine
- Cotton-wool balls
- Sterile drape
- Sterile gloves
- 20-ml syringe (for aspiration)
- 10-ml syringe (for local anaesthetic infiltration)
- Range of needle sizes
- 10 ml 1% lidocaine
- 3-way tap
- Luer lock syringe (50-ml)
- 18-gauge cannula
- Specimen bottles.

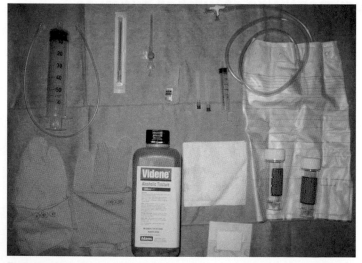

Equipment for pleural aspiration

ICE

- **I**ntroduce yourself.
- **C**onsent the patient for the procedure. Emphasise the risk of pneumothorax to the patient.
- **E**xpose the necessary part of the body and position the patient. This procedure should be undertaken with the patient sitting in a chair or on the edge of the bed leaning forwards. The arms should be crossed and supported by a pillow rested on a table or equivalent. This supports the weight of the arms allowing the upper body to be relaxed.

Procedure

- The correct location for the aspiration must be identified first. This may be found clinically or with radiological marking.
- Assess the most recent chest x-ray, coagulation screen and platelet count. Expert advice should be sought if any of these blood parameters are abnormal.
- The upper border of the effusion should be percussed (see page 13) in the mid-clavicular line posteriorly. Choose the intercostal space below the upper border of dullness and mark with an indelible marker.
- If the site has been radiologically marked, double-check the position with a clinical assessment before going ahead with the procedure.
- Wash your hands and put on sterile gloves.
- Request for each piece of the equipment to be handed to you in turn in an aseptic manner.
- Clean the chosen area with chlorhexidine and then iodine solution.
- Place a sterile drape over the posterior chest. This should have a ready-made hole in it so that the aspiration site can be visualised.
- Infiltrate the area for insertion of the needle with local anaesthetic. Use up to 5–10 ml of 1% lidocaine, initially as a bleb under the skin, and then deeper through subcutaneous tissues of the chest wall to the pleura. Insert the needle on the superior aspect of the rib to avoid the neurovascular bundle. Aspirate before injecting to ensure that the needle is not within a blood vessel. When the needle is far enough in, pleural fluid will be aspirated into the syringe, confirming correct location.
- Withdraw the needle, and cover the site temporarily with a piece of sterile gauze.

For diagnostic aspiration only

- Insert a new needle with an attached 20 ml syringe into the same spot as before.
- Aspirate the necessary pleural fluid volume for analysis.
- Withdraw the needle.
- Proceed to 'Completing the procedure'.

For therapeutic aspiration

- Familiarise yourself with the 3-way tap and Luer lock syringe. Adjust the 3-way tap so that it is closed.
- Attach the 50-ml syringe to the port of a cannula (at least 18-gauge).
- Using firm pressure, slowly pass the cannula through the anaesthetised area of skin, aspirating on the syringe at the same time. Continue until you can see the pleural fluid enter the syringe.
- Simultaneously insert the cannula while withdrawing the needle.
- Attach the 3-way tap to the cannula port. Attach the 50-ml syringe to the tap, and open the valve.
- Aspirate pleural fluid until the syringe is full. Close the tap, and discard the contents of the syringe.
- Repeat this until you have removed the necessary volume of fluid.
- For routine purposes, do not remove more than 1000 ml of pleural fluid on a single occasion.
- Withdraw the cannula.

Completing the procedure

- Place a piece of sterile gauze over the area of puncture and secure with tape.
- Place the pleural fluid into the necessary specimen bottles.
- Dispose of sharps carefully.
- Wash your hands.
- Order a check chest radiograph to exclude a pneumothorax.
- Document the procedure in the medical notes (as outlined below).
- Monitor the vital signs (especially SpO_2) regularly post procedure.

Always consider the risk of causing a pneumothorax.

Do not remove more than 1000 ml in a single aspiration.

Investigations of pleural fluid

- Cytology
- Culture (may include Mycobacterium species)
- Protein
- LDH
- Glucose
- pH
- Amylase
- Immunology (when indicated)
- Microscopy (white cell count)

Documentation of procedure

An accurate medical note is essential. For example:

28/06/2004, 10.15 hours, B. Stockham (PRHO)

Therapeutic and diagnostic pleural tap

- Indication: shortness of breath.
- Consent obtained
- Aseptic technique
- 5 ml of 1% lidocaine infiltration subcutaneously
- 18-gauge needle on first pass into 8th intercostal space, right side
- 440 ml of bloodstained fluid aspirated
- Sent for cytology, microbiology, LDH, glucose, protein content, pH and amylase
- Check chest x-ray requested.

For a peritoneal tap to be undertaken the patient must have ascites. This should be clinically detectable unless the procedure is to be carried out under imaging guidance.

The procedure may involve the aspiration of a small volume of ascitic fluid for diagnostic purposes. In other patients (especially those with recurrent ascites), larger volumes of fluid may be removed for therapeutic relief. In such circumstances huge volumes of fluid may have accumulated and aspiration should be performed cautiously. The patient should empty the bladder before the procedure to minimise the risk of bladder puncture. In some cases urinary catheterisation may be required. Therapeutic paracentesis is traditionally carried out using a 3-way tap syringe. Increasingly, the Bonnano catheter technique is being used. Both methods will be described in this section.

Equipment

- Dressing pack
- Antiseptic fluid (usually chlorhexidine) and iodine
- Cotton-wool balls
- Sterile drape
- Sterile gloves
- 20-ml syringe (for aspiration)
- 10-ml syringe (for local anaesthetic infiltration)
- Scalpel
- Range of needle sizes
- 5 ml of 1% lidocaine
- 3-way tap or Bonnano catheter kit (if therapeutic tap to be undertaken).

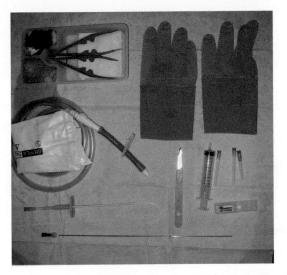

Equipment for peritoneal tap (paracentesis) – Bonnano catheter method

ICE

- **I**ntroduce yourself.
- **C**onsent the patient for the procedure.
- **E**xpose the necessary part of the body and position the patient. The patient should be supine, lying as flat as is tolerated. The hips should be extended. The entire abdomen should be exposed.

Procedure

- Assess a recent coagulation screen and platelet count. Expert advice should be sought if either of these parameters are abnormal.
- Assess the abdomen for shifting dullness (see page 22).
- Choose an appropriate location – usually in the left or right iliac fossa. In the case of tense ascites for therapeutic tap (by the bonnano catheter method), a site in the midline, 1cm inferior to the umbilicus, inferior may be used. Avoid any visible vessels on the abdominal wall.
- Wash your hands and put on sterile gloves.
- Request for each piece of the equipment to be handed to you in turn in an aseptic manner.
- Clean the chosen area with chlorhexidine and then iodine solution.
- Place a sterile drape over the abdomen. This should have a ready-made hole in it so that the aspiration site can be visualised.

- Infiltrate the chosen site with local anaesthetic. Use up to 5 ml of 1% lidocaine, initially as a bleb under the skin and then deeper through the abdominal wall. Aspirate before injecting to ensure that the needle is not within a blood vessel. With tense ascites, correct location is confirmed by peritoneal fluid being aspirated into the syringe.

For diagnostic aspiration only

- Leave the needle in situ and use a new 20 ml syringe to aspirate the necessary fluid volume for analysis.
- Withdraw the needle.
- Place a piece of sterile gauze over the puncture site, and tape in place.
- Proceed to 'Completing the procedure'.

For therapeutic paracentesis

Bonnano catheter method

- Remove the needle.
- Make a small (5mm) incision with the scalpel on the abdominal wall through the skin and subcutaneous tissue.
- Familiarise oneself with the bonnano catheter kit. This should contain a trochar with an overlying pigtail catheter. The catheter will be curled at this stage. Straighten it by passing the trochar to to the limit of the catheter.
- Using firm pressure pass the trochar through the skin incision using minimal force.
- Pass cautiously until a flash back of ascitic fluid is seen.
- At this point pass the catheter over the trochar into the abdomen, whilst withdrawing the trochar.
- When fully inserted, the retaining disc will abut the abdominal wall. With the trochar removed, the catheter will have curled up inside the abdomen, helping it to remain in place.

- Attach the collection bag to the catheter tubing and attach a clamp.
- Fix the end of the retaining disc tightly to the abdominal wall with cannula dressings. Alternatively, sutures can be used.
- Inform nursing staff how much fluid is to be removed. The clamp should be used if drainage is occurring too rapidly.

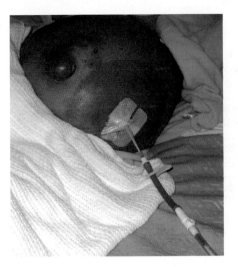

Therapeutic paracentesis – Bonnano catheter method

3-way tap method

- Familiarise yourself with the 3-way tap kit.
- Insert an 18- or 16-gauge cannula through the anaesthetised area of the abdominal wall.
- Pass the cannula cautiously until a flashback of ascitic fluid is seen. At this stage, withdraw the needle while simultaneously inserting the cannula.
- Attach a 3-way tap to the port on the cannula.
- Attach a 50 ml syringe to one of the ports on the tap, and a collection bag to the other port.
- Manipulating the 3-way-tap, aspirate 50 ml at a time from the abdomen into the syringe, and subsequently into the collection bag.
- Continue until the desired volume has been removed.

100 ml of intravenous 20% albumin should be infused for every 3 litres of ascitic fluid removed.

Completing the procedure

- Dispose of sharps carefully.
- Place ascitic fluid samples within specimen bottles for analysis.
- Wash your hands.
- Document the procedure in the medical notes (as outlined below).

The patient must have an empty bladder.

Assess the patient's coagulation status before the procedure.

Discontinue the procedure if the patient becomes hypotensive.

Investigations to be carried out on ascitic fluid

- Cytology
- Culture (microbiology)
- Microscopy (white cell count)
- Protein
- Amylase
- Glucose
- LDH

Documentation of peritoneal tap

An accurate medical note is essential. For example:

12/6/2004, 15.10 hours, C. Civil (SHO)

Therapeutic peritoneal tap

- Indication: recurrent ascites; hepatocellular carcinoma; tense ascites

- Consent obtained

- Coagulation status and platelet count normal

- Aseptic technique

- 5 ml of 1% lidocaine infiltrated subcutaneously

- 5mm incision made with scalpel

- Bonnano catheter inserted first pass

- Free flow of peritoneal fluid – straw-coloured

- To remain in situ for no more than 24 hours

- 100 ml of 20% albumin for each 3 litres removed

- No more than 2 litres per hour. Clamp if necessary.

SECTION 4
RADIOLOGY

Reading a chest radiograph

Technical aspects

Name and date of examination

Always check that it is the correct patient, and that it is the appropriately dated examination. (It is not uncommon for patients to have dozens of chest radiographs). This is sound practice for any radiographic examination.

Rotation

The spinous processes of the vertebrae should be equidistant from the medial borders of the clavicle.

Inspiration

There should be ten posterior ribs visible in the mid-clavicular line on full inspiration.

Penetration

The vertebral bodies should be visible through the heart shadow.

Review areas

These are structures that should be evaluated in every chest radiograph:

• Heart size and shape

• Pulmonary vasculature

• Lungs (including hila)

• Bony contours (ribs, spine, shoulders)

• Soft tissues (especially breast shadows, axillae and neck).

Don't relax on finding one abnormality. There may be more than one and the relationship may be clinically important (eg pleural effusion and mastectomy).

The normal cardiac outline

Cardiothoracic ratio

The maximum transverse diameter of the heart should not exceed 55% of the maximum transverse diameter of the chest.

Right heart border

This shadow is formed by (from above, downwards):

• Superior vena cava

• Right atrium

• Inferior vena cava.

Left heart border

This shadow is formed by (from above, downwards):

- Aortic knuckle
- Pulmonary trunk
- Left atrial appendage
- Left ventricle.

Normal pulmonary vascularity

Discrete vessels should not be visible in the outer third of the lung fields.

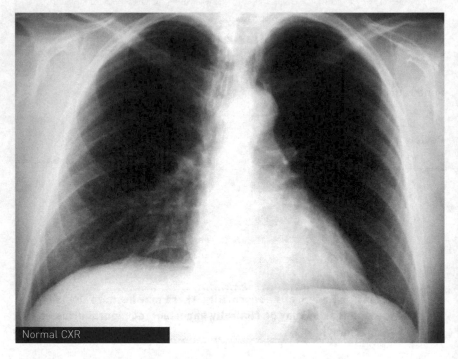

Normal CXR

Common chest radiograph abnormalities

Cardiac failure

Cardiothoracic ratio

The heart enlarges and the transverse diameter increases to > 55%.

Upward venous diversion

As cardiac decompensation occurs, there is upward shunting of blood so the vascularity increases. (Normally, a superior pulmonary vein, measured in the second interspace, measures < 2–3 mm.)

Pulmonary vascularity

Enlargement of the radiating vessels means that they are discretely visible in the outer third of the lung.

Kerley B lines

These are peripheral horizontal lines at the margins of the lung bases seen (but not exclusively) in cardiac failure.

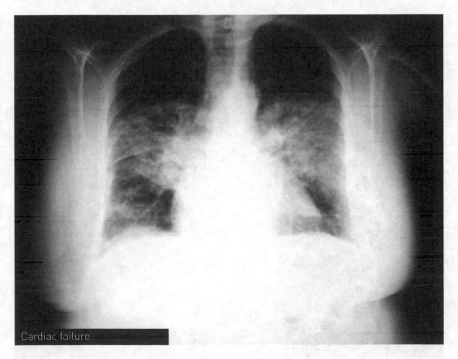

Cardiac failure

Air space change

As the pulmonary venous pressure increases to > 25 mmHg, pulmonary oedema occurs, and the acini become consolidated. At this stage, air bronchograms are identified, typically bilaterally and in a perihilar location (the so-called 'bat's wing' appearance).

Lobar pneumonia

The silhouette sign

This states that the heart shadow and the diaphragm are visible because they are surrounded by air in the surrounding pulmonary acini. If lobar consolidation occurs, the adjacent acini obscure that portion of the silhouette. The specific silhouette losses are described below for the associated lobar consolidations.

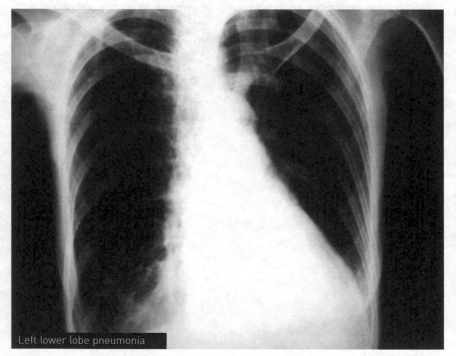

Left lower lobe pneumonia

Specific silhouette losses with associated lobar consolidations

- Right upper lobe   Right upper mediastinum
- Right middle lobe   Right heart border
- Right lower lobe   Right hemidiaphragm
- Left upper lobe   Aortic knuckle
- Lingula   Left heart border
- Left lower lobe   Left hemidiaphragm

With ensuing lobar collapse there is:

- Volume loss (ipsilateral)
- Diaphragmatic elevation
- Movement of the ipsilateral hilum towards the collapsed lobe.

Pulmonary mass lesion

One can localise perihilar lesions by using the silhouette sign. Lesions in the middle mediastinum will obscure the adjacent heart or mediastinal shadow. Lesions in front of or behind the heart will allow the cardiac and mediastinal shadows to be identified despite the discrete lesion.

Lesions above the clavicle on the frontal chest radiograph are posteriorly placed. (Always look for associated posterior rib erosion or destruction.)

Lesions by location

Anterior mediastinal mass

- Thymic tumours
- Teratoma
- Lymphoma
- Retrosternal thyroid

Middle mediastinal mass

- Bronchogenic carcinoma
- Lymphadenopathy
- Aortic aneurysm

Posterior mediastinal mass

- Aortic aneurysm
- Neurogenic tumours
- Paravertebral abscesses
- Dilated oesophagus

Pneumothorax

This is more easily demonstrated in the expiratory phase, when the relatively positive intrapleural pressure pushes the lung edge away from the chest wall. The lung edge is demonstrated against the relative 'blackness' of the intrapleural air.

Tension pneumothorax

If there is a valve type effect, eg following a stabbing, with each breath more air is introduced into the pleural space, and the lung becomes progressively pushed away from the chest wall.

Signs of tension

- Flattening or depression of the ipsilateral hemidiaphragm
- Movement of the medistinum to the contralateral side.

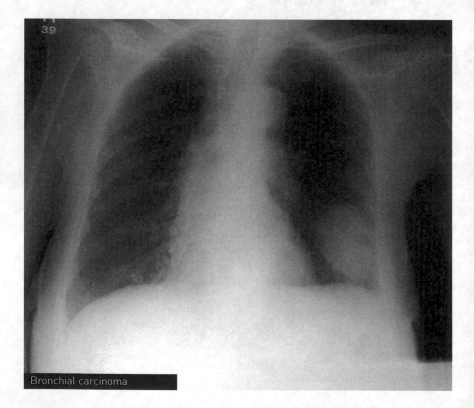

Bronchial carcinoma

Pleural effusion

Loss of basal aerated lung means that there is usually loss of the hemidiaphragm's silhouette on the erect radiograph. In addition, the fluid curves upwards peripherally at the lung edge to produce a crescentic meniscus. Mass effect will displace the heart to the contralateral side (unless there is associated lobar collapse, when the mass effect of the effusion is 'neutralised' by the volume loss of the collapsed lung lobe).

In the supine film, look for a veiled, greying of the affected side, caused by fluid lying posteriorly between the lung and the chest wall. This is a particularly crucial observation to make in an emergency trauma patient, who may have substantial volume of blood concealed in the intrapleural space.

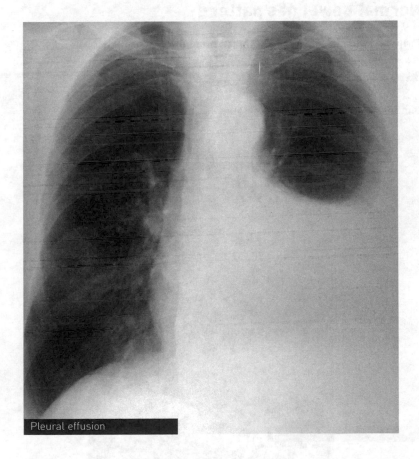

Pleural effusion

A structured approach for inspection of the abdominal radiograph will aid assessment. A framework as detailed below is advised.

> **Points to be inspected on every abdominal radiograph**
> - Technical aspects
> - Intraluminal gas
> - Extraluminal gas
> - Calcification
> - Bones and soft tissues
> - Iatrogenic, accidental and incidental objects

Normal bowel gas pattern

Proportion of gas within the stomach and bowel
- Normally gas in stomach, colon and rectum
- There is little gas in the small bowel.

Dimensions of the jejunum and ileum
- Wall thickness: 2–2.5 mm
- Lumen diameter: 2–3 cm.

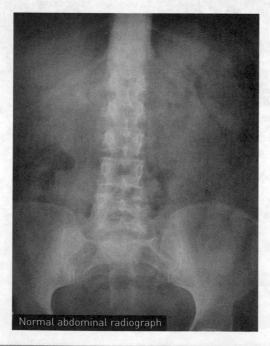

Normal abdominal radiograph

Common abdominal radiograph abnormalities

Intestinal obstruction

Small-bowel obstruction

- Distended bowel centrally
- Valvulae conniventes present
- Diameter < 5cm.

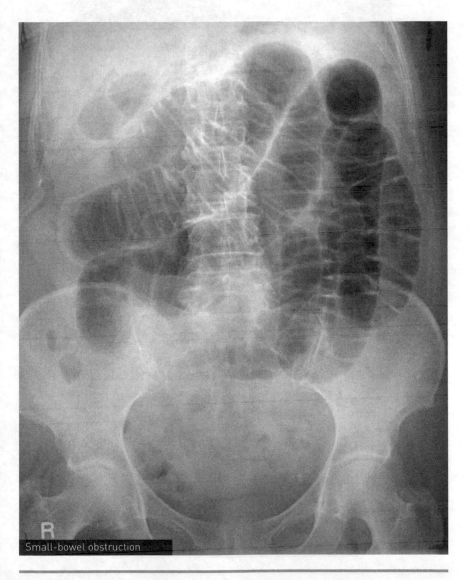

Small-bowel obstruction

Large-bowel obstruction

- Distended bowel peripherally
- Haustra, but no valvulae
- Diameter > 5 cm.

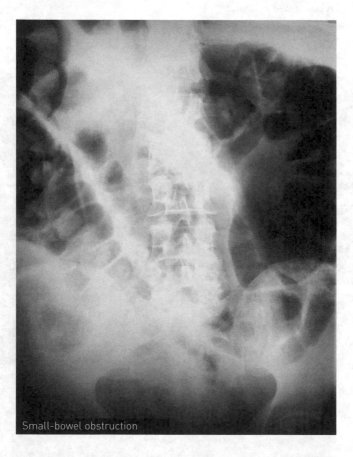

Small-bowel obstruction

Volvulus

Any portion of bowel on a mesentery may twist about that mesentery to produce a volvulus. Caecal and sigmoid volvuli are most common, although a gastric volvulus may occur.

Caecal volvulus

- Single enlarged loop
- Mostly fluid-filled (high fluid:air ratio)
- No gas in large bowel
- Younger age group (30–40 years).

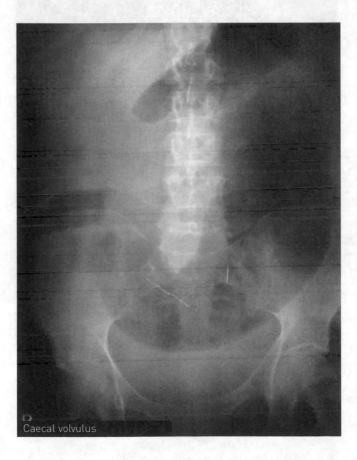

Caecal volvulus

Sigmoid volvulus

- Two loops (coffee-bean sign)
- Mostly air-filled (low fluid:air ratio)
- Distended large bowel
- Tapered sigmoid obstruction ('bird of prey' sign)
- Older age group (> 60 years).

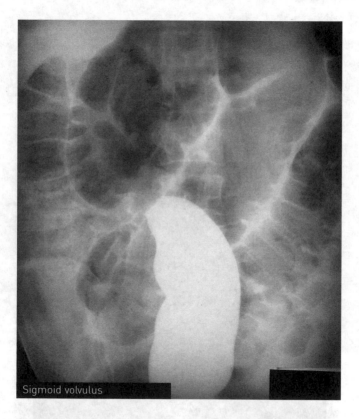

Sigmoid volvulus

Ileus and pseudo-obstruction

These can be differentated from mechanical bowel obstruction.

Intestinal obstruction

- Abdominal pain
- Gas-filled bowel loops
- Cut-off point.

Ileus

- No abdominal pain
- Gas-filled bowel loops
- No cut-off point.

Pseudo-obstruction

- Abdominal pain
- Gas-filled bowel loops
- No cut-off point
- Differential caecal enlargement.

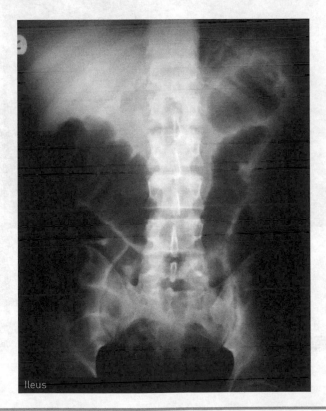

Ileus

Pneumoperitoneum

The erect abdominal radiograph

- Free air under diaphragm (right side more sensitive than left).

The supine abdominal radiograph

- Rigler's sign (free air on both sides of the bowel wall)
- Falciform ligament sign (the sickle-shaped falciform ligament is outlined by air in a band running between the liver and the umbilicus).

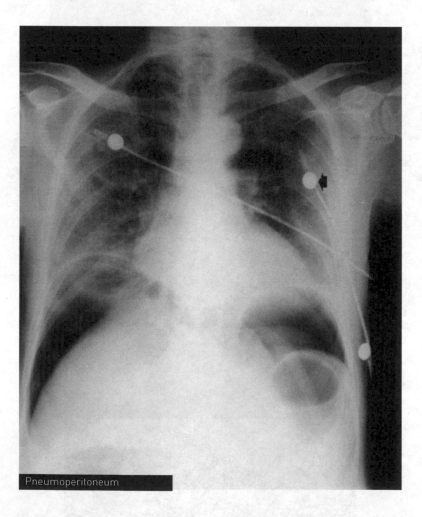

Pneumoperitoneum

Inflammatory bowel disease

Toxic megacolon

- Widening of the transverse colonic lumen (> 5.5 cm)
- Mucosal oedema (thumb-printing)
- No residual faecal shadows (catharsis).

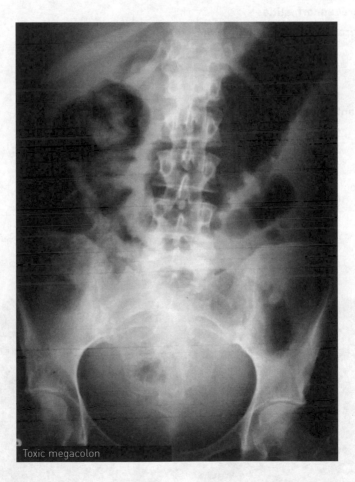

Toxic megacolon

Miscellaneous

Hepatomegaly

- Descent of right lobe into the right iliac fossa
- Beware Riedel's lobe – true hepatomegaly has enlargement of both lobes; Riedel's lobe typically has a normal or small left lobe.

Vertebral abnormalities

Degeneration (spondylosis)

- Reduction of disc space
- Osteophytes at bony margins
- Sclerotic bony margins.

Malignant infiltration

- Check that both pedicles are present at each vertebral level.
- Malignant infiltration destroys the pedicle first and may be seen as an absent pedicle, giving the appearance of a 'winking eye'.

Pathological calcification

Chronic pancreatitis
Flecks of calcification transversely across the upper abdomen in chronic pancreatitis (30–40%). (Calcification is rare in adenocarcinoma of the pancreas – only 2% of cases.)

Calcification of the renal parenchyma may occur – this is nephrocalcinosis.

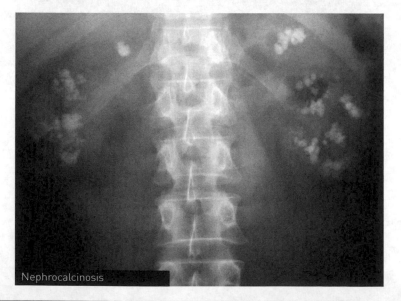

Nephrocalcinosis

Aortic aneurysm
- A convex arc of calcification, aligned with the vertebral column.
- The calcification is on the endothelial surface, and therefore indicates the 'inner' diameter of the aneurysm.
- Better appreciated on the lateral X-ray.

Key Terms

Contralateral: opposite side

Crescentic: shaped like a crescent or half-moon

Equidistant: equal distance between two objects or places

Hemidiaphragm: half of the diaphragm

Intrapleural: within the pleura

Ipsilateral: same side

Lingula: superior and inferior bronchopulmonary segments, generally considered to be part of the left upper lobe

Perihilar: around the hilar region of the lung

Transverse diameter of chest: distance between the midline and the outermost limit of the thoracic cavity (measured at the widest point)

INDEX

Page numbers in *italics* refer to diagrams and radiographs

N O T E S

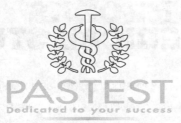

DEDICATED TO YOUR SUCCESS

PasTest has been publishing books for medical students and doctors for over 30 years. Our extensive experience means that we are always one step ahead when it comes to knowledge of current trends in undergraduate exams.

We use only the best authors, which enables us to tailor our books to meet your revision needs. We incorporate feedback from candidates to ensure that our books are continually improved.

This commitment to quality ensures that students who buy PasTest books achieve successful exam results.

Delivery to your door
With a busy lifestyle, nobody enjoys walking to the shops for something that may or may not be in stock. Let us take the hassle and deliver direct to your door. We will dispatch your book within 24 hours of receiving your order.

How to Order:
www.pastest.co.uk
To order books safely and securely online, shop at our website.

Telephone: +44 (0)1565 752000   Fax: +44 (0)1565 650264
For priority mail order and have your credit card to hand when you call.

Write to us at:
PasTest Ltd
FREEPOST
Haig Road
Parkgate Industrial Estate
Knutsford
WA16 7BR

PASTEST BOOKS
FOR MEDICAL STUDENTS

PasTest are the specialists in study guides and revision courses for medical qualifications. For over 30 years we have been helping doctors to achieve their potential. The PasTest range of books for medical students includes:

Essential Skills Practice for OSCEs in Medicine   1 904627 38 2
David McCluskey

100 Clinical Cases and OSCEs in Medicine   1 904627 12 9
David McCluskey

100 Clinical Cases and OSCEs in Surgery   1 904627 00 5
Arnold Hill, Noel Aherne

OSCEs for Medical Students, Volume 1   1 904627 09 9
Adam Feather, Ramanathan Visvanathan,
John SP Lumley

OSCEs for Medical Students, Volume 2   1 904627 10 2
Adam Feather, Ramanathan Visvananthan,
John SP Lumley

OSCEs for Medical Students, Volume 3   1 904627 11 0
Adam Feather, Ramanathan Visvananthan,
John SP Lumley, Jonathan Round

EMQs for Medical Students, Volume 1   1 901198 65 0
Adam Feather et al

EMQs for Medical Students, Volume 2   1 901198 69 3
Adam Feather et al

EMQs for Medical Students, Volume 3
Practice Papers   1 904627 07 2
Adam Feather et al